AT YOUR FINGE

HIGH
BLOOD PRESSURE

THIRD EDITION

Tom Fahey MSc, MD, MFPHM, MRCGP
Professor of Primary Care Medicine,
Tayside Centre of General Practice, University of Dundee;
General Practitioner at Taybank Medical Practice, Dundee

with a chapter on high blood pressure in pregnancy by

Deirdre Murphy MD MRCOG
Professor of Obstetrics, University of Dundee;
Consultant Obstetrician, Ninewells Hospital, Dundee

Julian Tudor Hart MB, BChir, DCH, FRCP, FRCGP
Honorary Research Fellow at Welsh Institute for Health
and Social Care, University of Glamorgan, Pontypridd

CLASS PUBLISHING • LONDON

Printing history
First published 1996
Reprinted 1997
Reprinted with revisions 1997
Second edition 1999
Reprinted 2000
Reprinted 2001
Reprinted 2002
Reprinted 2003
Third edition 2004

The authors and publishers welcome feedback from the users of this book. Please contact the publishers.

**Class Publishing (London) Ltd, Barb House, Barb Mews,
London W6 7PA
Telephone: 020 7371 2119
Fax: 020 7371 2878 [International +4420]
email: post@class.co.uk
Visit our website – www.class.co.uk**

The information presented in this book is accurate and current to the best of the authors' knowledge. The authors and publisher, however, make no guarantee as to, and assume no responsibility for, the correctness, sufficiency or completeness of such information or recommendation. The reader is advised to consult a doctor regarding all aspects of individual health care.

A CIP catalogue record for this book is available from the British Library

ISBN 1 85959 090 X

Edited by Susan Bosanko and Michèle Clarke (1st and 2nd editions), Michèle Clarke (3rd edition)

Indexed by Michèle Clarke

Cartoons by Julian Tudor Hart

Line illustrations by David Woodroffe

Typeset by Martin Bristow

Printed and bound in Finland by WS Bookwell, Juva

Comments on High Blood Pressure – the 'at your fingertips' guide *from readers*

'... readable and comprehensive information for anyone with high blood pressure ...'

Dr Sylvia McLauchlan MB, ChB, MSc, FFPHM
Former Director General, The Stroke Association

'It is very readable, I think pitched at just the right level.'

Professor Godfrey Fowler
Emeritus Professor of General Practice, University of Oxford

'I have thoroughly enjoyed reading this book, it has covered all the questions that I and most people especially those with high blood pressure would like to ask.'

Evelyn Thomas SRN, Glyncorrwg

'This book answers the questions you always wanted to ask about high blood pressure, plus many you haven't even thought of.'

Gwen Hall RMN, RGN, BSc, Hindhead

'I have enjoyed reading *High Blood Pressure – the 'at your fingertips' guide* and now feel much better informed.

Mrs Shirley Wallwork

'... a clear and comprehensive review of hypertension, its causes, clinical picture and treatment. A must for the bookshelf of all those interested in, or suffering from, high blood pressure.'

H. Rees, Killay

'I have always been health conscious and a believer in taking control of my own health. When I was told by my GP that I had high blood pressure, I wanted to find out everything I could about it before starting any treatment. This book has not disappointed me – it has answered all my questions, and I now feel more confident about arranging a suitable treatment plan with my GP.'

Andrea Bagg, Tunbridge Wells

'This is a really excellent book and a very valuable addition to the series.'

Professor Paul Wallace, Royal Free Hospital School of Medicine

'As someone who has had high blood pressure for 29 years I still found this book enlightening and was impressed by the fact that I felt because of the way the author had written the book that it was really speaking to me, and as a result I didn't find it wearisome reading like some information books.'

Babs Walters, Port Talbot

'The language is pitched at just the right level so that the reader feels he has been taken into partnership with the doctor in understanding his condition.'

Dr A. G. Donald, Edinburgh

'Exactly the right style for dealing with the sort of problems that patients regularly have. It is not only educational but extremely enjoyable.'

Professor John Swales, Professor of Medicine, University of Leicester

Reviews of **High Blood Pressure – the 'at your fingertips' guide**

'This well written book is capable of informing health professionals . . . The question and answer format of the book gives comprehensive coverage.'

Adrienne Willcox, Practice Nurse

'Dr Julian Tudor Hart has produced an excellent book . . . with a comprehensive question and answer format which will solve any query.'

Dr Donald McKendrick, Saga Magazine

Contents

Acknowledgements

We should like to thank our colleagues at Taybank Medical Practice, Dundee, and the Department of Obstetrics and Gynaecology and the Cardiovascular Risk Clinic at Ninewells Hospital, Dundee, for their continuing support. Professor Mark Caulfield (St Bartholomew's and The London, Queen Mary's School of Medicine) provided additional material relating to genetics and high blood pressure for which we are grateful. Thanks also to Debbie O'Farrell for administrative support and our colleagues at Tayside Centre for General Practice and the Division of Maternal and Child Health Sciences, University of Dundee. Michèle Clarke provided excellent editorial guidance. We should like to thank Dr Philip Kell, author of *Sexual Health for Men – the 'at your fingertips' guide*, for providing a question on sex and high blood pressure.

Our largest debt of gratitude is to Professors Julian Tudor Hart and Wendy Savage, who wrote the original edition of this book. This third edition has been modified to reflect the recent evidence concerning detection, treatment and management of high blood pressure. However, large parts of the text have remained unaltered, a tribute to the original work done by Julian and Wendy. We alone are responsible for any errors in the text.

Foreword

by Dr Julian Hart

MB, BChir, DCH, FRCP, FRCGP

High blood pressure is the most common continuing medical condition seen by family doctors. At just what measurement 'normal' blood pressure becomes 'high' blood pressure that justifies action being taken to reduce it is still a subject for professional argument among doctors (although most now agree on a pressure of somewhere around 160/90 mmHg). Whatever the definition, the numbers of people needing some sort of treatment for high blood pressure include at least 10% of any large group of adults, up to 33% of poorer city adults, and about 50% of all people over 65 years of age – a lot of people.

If you are one of this 10–50%, and you need medication for your high blood pressure, you will probably go on needing it for the rest of your life. If you read, understand, and remember the following few pages, you will be well on the way to understanding the nature of your high blood pressure, what can and what can't be done about it, and both the benefits and risks of treatment. If not, your alternative is to let doctors take decisions about your life, without your help or informed consent. Most doctors today understand how dangerous it is for the people they treat to be so uninformed and uncritical. Safe doctoring depends on the cooperative work of two sets of experts: expert professionals who know a lot about how the human body works but little about the personal lives of the people they are treating; and the people being treated, who are experts on their own lives but know rather less about how their bodies work. Just as doctors can't look after you properly if they are completely ignorant of your life, so you can't interpret their advice safely if you are completely ignorant of human biology.

Even if you remember only these few pages, you will know more about the practical management of high blood pressure than many health professionals, who usually have to cover a much wider range of medical conditions and cannot concentrate only on this one. With or without this knowledge, you, not your doctors, will be responsible for actually using the treatments they recommend. Many different drugs are used to treat high blood pressure, but they all have one thing in common: they don't work if you don't take them. Yet many (if not most) people treated for high blood pressure don't take their tablets regularly. They take them if they feel as though their blood pressure is high, but miss them if they feel well or plan to have a few drinks, or need to take other tablets for something else and are afraid of mixing them, or if they're afraid of side-effects and even more afraid of admitting this to their doctor. Unless you are in hospital you have to take your own treatment decisions – there are no nurses' rounds to see that you follow orders. To medicate yourself safely you need far more information than any doctor or nurse can impart in the few minutes usually available for a consultation, and one purpose of this book is to provide you with that information.

What high blood pressure is and what it is not

Everybody's blood is under pressure, otherwise it wouldn't circulate around the body. If blood pressure is too high it damages the walls of your arteries. After many years, this damage increases your risks of coronary heart disease, heart failure, stroke, bleeding or detachment of the retina (the back of the eye), and kidney failure. High blood pressure itself is not a disease, but a treatable cause of these serious diseases, which are thereby partly preventable. All these risks are greatly increased if you also smoke or have diabetes.

Unless it has already caused damage, high BP seldom makes you feel unwell. It can be very high without causing headaches, breathlessness, palpitations, faintness, giddiness, or any of the symptoms which were once thought to be typical of high BP. You may have any or all of these symptoms without having high BP, and you may have dangerously high BP with none of them.

The only way to know if you have high blood pressure (and how high it is) is to measure it with an instrument called a sphygmomanometer while you are sitting quietly. Because BP varies so much from hour to hour and from day to day, this should be done at least three times (preferably on separate days) to work out a true average figure before you take big decisions like starting or stopping treatment.

Mechanisms

Your level of BP depends on how hard your heart pumps blood into your arteries, on the volume of blood in your circulation, and on how tight your arteries are. The smaller arteries are sheathed by a strand of muscle which spirals around them: if this muscle tightens and shortens, it narrows the artery. In this way smaller arteries can be varied in diameter according to varying needs of different organs in different activities. In people with high BP something goes wrong with this mechanism, so that all the arteries are too tight. The heart then has to beat harder to push blood through them. This tightening-up may be caused by signals sent by the brain through the nervous system, or by chemical signals (hormones) released by other organs in the body (such as the kidneys).

Causes

The causes of short-term rises in blood pressure which last only seconds or minutes are well understood, but these are not what we normally mean by high blood pressure. High blood pressure is important only when it is maintained for months or years – it is a high average pressure which is significant, not occasional high peaks. The causes of a long-term rise in average pressure are not fully known, but we do know that it runs in families. This inherited tendency seems to account for about half the differences between people; the rest seems to depend on how they live and what they eat (not just in adult life, but what they ate in infancy and childhood and how well-nourished they were before they were born). We don't know enough about this to be able to prevent most cases.

One cause we do know about is overweight (particularly in young people) and weight reduction is a sensible first step in treatment. Weight loss depends mainly on using up more energy (measured in calories) by taking more exercise, and reducing energy input (the number of calories eaten in food). In practice the most healthy way to do this is by reducing the amount of fats, oils, meat, sugar and alcohol in the diet, and instead eating more fruit, vegetables, cereal foods and fish (some of these foods have other good effects as well as helping weight loss). Eating less fat and oil is by far the most important of these changes. Another benefit from these changes in diet is that they help lower blood cholesterol levels and so reduce the risk of developing coronary heart disease.

Another known cause is excessive alcohol (which means **more than 4 units of alcohol a day for a man or 3 units a day for a woman – a unit of alcohol is one glass of wine or one single measure of spirits or half a pint of average strength beer or lager**). Again, the biggest effect is in young people. Limiting alcohol intake often brings high BP back to normal without any other treatment.

Stress

If you are anxious, angry, have been hurrying, have a full bladder or if you are cold then your BP will rise for a few minutes or even a few hours (so BP measured at such times is not reliable) – but none of these things seem to be causes of permanently raised blood pressure. High blood pressure seems to be just as common in peaceable, even-tempered people without worries as it is in excitable people with short fuses. However, feeling pushed at work or at home may be an important cause in some people, if not for everyone.

The word 'hypertension' is used in medical jargon with exactly the same meaning as high blood pressure. This does not mean that feeling tense necessarily raises blood pressure, nor does it mean that most people with high blood pressure feel tense. Blood pressure falls considerably during normal sleep, both in people with normal blood pressure and in those whose blood pressure is high. Training in relaxation certainly lowers blood pressure for a while, and may have a useful long-term effect on high blood pressure in people who learn how to switch off often during the day, but there is no evidence that treatment by relaxation alone is an effective or safe alternative to drug treatment for people with severe high blood pressure.

Salt and sodium

Table salt is sodium chloride: it is the sodium which is important for your blood pressure, not the chloride. High blood pressure is unknown among those peoples of the world whose normal diet contains about 20 times less sodium than a normal Western diet, and even very high BP can be controlled by reducing sodium intake to this low level. The diet required for this consists entirely of rice, fruit and vegetables and would be intolerable to most people in this country.

The usual British diet contains much more salt than anyone needs. It certainly does no harm to reduce sodium intake by not adding salt to cooked meals, and by reducing or avoiding high sodium processed foods (crisps, sausages, sauces, tinned meats and beans, and 'convenience' foods generally), Chinese take-aways (which contain huge quantities of sodium glutamate) and strong cheeses. Salt can be found in the most unexpected foods – for example, both milk and bread contain salt in amounts which would surprise most people.

There is no convincing evidence that the roughly one-third reduction in sodium intake you can achieve by these **dietary** changes is an effective alternative to drug treatment for severe high blood pressure. Reducing fat in your diet by about a quarter reduces the potential complications of high blood pressure much more effectively than reducing your salt intake by about half. Most people find it difficult to reduce fat and salt at the same time, and fat reduction deserves a higher priority (especially as cutting down on fats will help you lose weight). However, people whose blood pressure is high enough for them to need to take drugs for it may manage on lower doses of their tablets if they reduce their sodium intake, and very heavy salt-eaters should try to cut down.

Smoking

Smoking is not a cause of high blood pressure, but it enormously increases the risks associated with it. If you have high blood pressure already, then if you also smoke you are three times more likely to have a heart attack than non-smokers if you are under 50 years old, and twice as likely to have one if you are over 50. Heart attacks in people under 45, and in women at all ages, happen much more frequently in smokers.

Smoking is a powerful risk factor in its own right, not only for coronary heart disease and stroke, but also for cancer of the mouth, nose, throat, lung, bladder and pancreas, and for asthma and other lung diseases. Unlike all other risk factors, it also affects your colleagues, family and friends (through passive smoking and the example you set to your children) and it costs a lot of money you could spend better in other ways.

When to have drug treatment

You will probably be advised to have drug treatment for your high blood pressure if there is already evidence of damage to your arteries, brain, heart, eyes or kidneys, or if you also have diabetes As a very rough guide, drug treatment is otherwise rarely justified unless your average blood pressure (averaged from at least three readings on separate days) is at least 160/100 mmHg. While you don't need to know exactly what these figures mean, you should know what they are in your own case, just as you do your own height and weight.

This threshold figure (plus or minus 5 mmHg either way) is based on evidence from large controlled trials in Britain, Australia, Scandinavia and the USA, which have shown worthwhile saving of life in many thousands of people. The benefits of drug treatment are greatest in the people with the highest pressures, or those who already have evidence of organ damage. Most of the benefit has been in reducing strokes, heart failure and kidney damage; the effects on coronary heart attacks have been much smaller (more important ways to prevent heart attacks are to stop smoking, maintain regular exercise, and stick to a diet low in saturated fats).

Blood pressure-lowering drugs

When severe high blood pressure is reduced by drugs, people live longer than if they are left untreated. Their treatment will not affect how they feel – it seldom makes people feel better, and they may sometimes even feel worse. The aim of all present treatments for high blood pressure is not to cure it, but to prevent its consequences by keeping pressure down to a safer level (whatever the underlying causes of high blood pressure are, they seem almost always to be permanent and are not affected by any of the treatments now available). Treatment must therefore nearly always continue for life – if you stop taking your tablets, your blood pressure will probably rise again, although this may take several months.

Unfortunately, all the drugs used for high blood pressure can cause unpleasant side effects in some people, although the newer blood pressure lowering drugs are generally easier to live with than the older ones. If you think your drugs are upsetting you, then say so, as there are alternatives. With so many blood pressure-lowering drugs now available your doctor should be able to tailor an individual treatment for you that minimizes side effects or even eliminates them altogether. Included among the side effects of blood pressure-lowering drugs are tiredness, depression and failure of erection: if any of these happen to you, then tell your doctor or nurse, as if they really are caused by your drugs, they will clear up soon after your medication is changed.

If you have any wheezing or asthma, then some blood pressure-lowering drugs can be very dangerous, so make sure your doctor knows about this. Some drugs used for back and joint pains can interfere with the effect of drugs given for high blood pressure, and you should ask your doctor about these if you take them. (Don't try to alter your medication yourself.) The contraceptive pill occasionally raises blood pressure very seriously, so women with high blood pressure should discuss other methods of birth control.

Remembering to take tablets is difficult for many people. Take them at set times, and ask your partner or a friend to help you learn the habit of regular medication. Don't stop taking your tablets just because you're going out for a drink – all blood pressure-lowering drugs can be taken with moderate amounts of alcohol.

Follow-up

Always bring all your tablets (not just those for your high BP) with you in their original containers when you see your doctor or nurse for follow-up, so that they know exactly what you are taking. If your blood pressure doesn't fall despite apparently adequate medication, think about your weight or your alcohol intake. Follow-up visits should be frequent at first, perhaps once a week until your blood pressure is controlled to under 160/90 mmHg. After that most doctors will want to check your blood pressure every three months or so; never go longer than six months without a check.

The end of the beginning

All this (and I mean all) is the least you need to know to take an intelligent share in responsibility for your future health, not just as a passive consumer of medical care, but as an active producer of better health (as everyone should be). However, I hope by now you are interested enough to want to know more than this. The rest of this book will tell you a lot more both of what we do know about high blood pressure and – just as important – what we don't know.

About this book

Most of you reading this will have been told that either you, or someone in your family, has raised blood pressure. The questions in this book are those asked by people like you every day; the answers are intended to help you be as informed as possible about your own care so that your treatment will be more successful and you will feel more in control. Remember that no one involved in this subject (including doctors and nurses) ever stops learning more about it. In fact, a few of you may read this book not because of your own health problems, but because in your work you are concerned with the health problems of other people.

Because different people have different requirements for information about high blood pressure, this book has been designed in a way that means you do not have to read it from cover to cover unless you wish to do so. The questions are arranged into chapters and sections, so you may care to dip into it in sections at a time, or look for the answer to a particular question by using the table of contents and the index. Cross-references in the text will lead you to more detailed information where this might be helpful, and essential information is repeated wherever it seems to be necessary. Having said all this, the book begins with a brief general outline of high blood pressure – **What you most need to know in 11 questions**. However much you dip into and skip through the rest of the book, may we ask you please to read these few pages thoroughly?

Not everyone will agree with every answer we have given, but future editions of this book can only be improved if you let us know where you disagree, or have found the advice to have been unhelpful, or if you have any questions which you think we have not covered. Please write to us c/o Class Publishing, Barb House, Barb Mews, London W6 7PA.

And finally, what are giraffes doing in this book? Obviously more pressure is needed to push blood up than to push it down. The animals which have to cope with the biggest changes in blood pressure are therefore giraffes, whose brain capillary blood pressure has to be kept constant whether their heads are six feet or so below their hearts (as when they drink) or six feet above them (when they eat leaves off trees). For this reason, a giraffe graces each chapter of this book, in an effort to reassure you that it is not unreadable.

Introduction
What you most need to know in 11 questions

What is high blood pressure (BP)?

High BP is not an illness or disease – rather it is a risk marker for illnesses that you wish to avoid. These include stroke, heart attacks, kidney problems and other problems affecting the circulatory system (blood circulation). Most people who have high BP do not have any symptoms. However, not having symptoms does not imply that you are not at risk of having any of the potentially harmful consequences of having high BP. The risk of suffering complications from having high BP can be reduced by either non-drug or drug treatments or by both.

What types of high BP are there?

High BP is traditionally classified into two main groups: 'essential' or primary hypertension where no cause can be found and 'secondary' hypertension where high BP is caused by other conditions. ('Hypertension' is just a medical name for high BP.)

Secondary hypertension is very uncommon and mostly caused by various sorts of kidney disease, or occasionally by irregular anatomy of the aorta ('coarctation'); overproduction of some BP-raising hormones by tumours of the pituitary gland, adrenal glands or kidneys; or by disorders involving compression of the brain. These 'classical' secondary causes altogether account for less than 1% of all treated cases of high BP.

1

What causes high BP?

There is still a lot of uncertainty about the causes of high BP. For the vast majority of people, over 95%, an underlying cause is not found. These are the people who have 'essential' hypertension. It is likely that several factors contribute to high BP in most people. The chief suspects include:

- an overactive hormone system that relates to the kidney (the renin–angiotensin system);
- an overactive autonomic nervous system (the part of the nervous system responsible for our unconscious nervous responses);
- a fault in the cells of the smaller blood vessels that produce substances leading to blood vessel narrowing and increased BP (endothelial cell dysfunction);
- genetic predisposition (when you may have inherited a tendency to high BP);
- intrauterine factors, particularly birth weight, that may reflect undernourishment in the fetus, and that 'programme' our body to develop high BP in later life.

How is high BP measured?

Accurate BP measurement is important for diagnosis. Raised BP is a symptomless condition that, if left untreated, contributes to a substantial risk of heart disease and stroke. Clinical trials of BP-lowering drugs have shown that reducing BP reduces the risk of heart disease and stroke.

BP can be measured in several ways: by means of an electronic, mercury or aneroid sphygmomanometer. Electronic monitors are being increasingly used in GPs' surgeries. Provided that a machine is selected that has been shown to be accurate and reliable, electronic monitoring offers several advantages over the older mercury sphygomanometers. Aneroid sphygmomanometers are unreliable and are not recommended.

How many readings and visits are needed before high BP is diagnosed?

There is no universally accepted number of visits that are necessary for a doctor to make a firm diagnosis of high BP. However, all national guidelines recommend multiple visits and multiple readings before high BP is diagnosed. Clinical trials that have established the benefits of BP-lowering treatments generally used two or three BP readings on two or more clinic visits to confirm a diagnosis. A minimum of three BP readings per visit over at least four or more separate visits are needed to confirm a diagnosis of hypertension.

What is white coat hypertension?

This is when your BP is high when measured during a surgery or outpatient clinic but is otherwise normal. It usually occurs in response to the measurement of BP by a doctor or nurse. In people with normal BP, there is generally little or no difference between their BP reading at a clinic or in a surgery compared to their usual BP reading. However, in some people, substantial differences between clinic and usual BP are consistently found, with the higher readings occurring in situations where a doctor or nurse has made the BP reading. This phenomenon of 'white coat hypertension' is more commonly seen in women and older people.

As many as 20% of people diagnosed with high BP at clinics or in surgery may have entirely normal BPs when it is measured during the rest of the day. Other BP measuring techniques are recommended in these people so that their usual pressure is accurately recorded.

Why do some people have their BP measured with a portable machine?

What you are describing is 'ambulatory' BP monitoring. Ambulatory BP monitoring is a much better way of measuring BP in somebody who has one of the following factors:

- white coat hypertension
- unusual variability in the measurement of BP at the clinic;
- 'uncontrolled hypertension' – this is high BP that has not been reduced to a target BP level after intensive drug treatment has been given;
- very low BP, particularly after suddenly standing up when someone may feel dizzy or light-headed (postural hypotension); in more severe cases this can cause fainting or a fall.

What tests might I need if I suffer from high BP?

The 'classical' causes of secondary high BP are all rare, accounting for less than 1% of all cases of treated high BP. In practice this means that detailed tests are not usually necessary when high BP is first diagnosed. The following are usually performed by your GP:

- *Urine test* to check for protein and sugar in the urine. Leakage of protein may indicate that the kidneys have been damaged from high BP and you will need more detailed assessment of your kidney function. Testing for sugar is a relatively straightforward way of checking for diabetes. Similarly, if sugar is present, then blood tests will be needed to confirm or rule out diabetes.
- *Blood tests* for urea, electrolytes and creatinine levels; total cholesterol/HDL cholesterol.

What about other risk factors? Do they need to be measured when considering treatment for high BP?

It is now recognized that high BP should not be seen and treated as a single risk factor. Guidelines now recommend that the choice of treatment depends on a person's 'cardiovascular' risk (your risk of suffering a stroke or heart attack). To assess your cardiovascular risk, the doctor will take any factors into account, such as age, sex, history of diabetes, whether you smoke or not, cholesterol levels, family history and past history of cardiovascular disease. Charts that place people into levels of cardiovascular risk have now been published, and many general practitioners use these charts to assess a person's risk of stroke or heart attack. Examples of these risk charts are included in Appendix 1.

A consequence of taking all these factors into account is that treatment recommendations are likely to include non-drug solutions, such as taking more exercise or stopping smoking. It also means that different types of drug treatments can be considered by your doctor, such as cholesterol-lowering drugs, BP-lowering drugs and drugs that prevent clotting (aspirin).

What are the best treatments without resorting to drugs?

The best thing you can do is to change your lifestyle: altering your diet, doing exercise and stopping smoking will lower the many risks that can cause high BP or that can increase you cardio-vascular risk level.

Increasing exercise, losing weight, lowering alcohol consumption and changing your diet (reducing salt intake and increasing fruit and vegetable intake) will result in a reduction of about 4 mmHg systolic BP on average if you stick to these changes. Though these falls in BP are not as substantial as drug treatment, other risk factors will be improved at the same time, resulting in an overall reduction of your cardiovascular risk. Such changes are also highly beneficial in older patients as well.

Lastly, if you are a smoker, stopping smoking is the most effective way of reducing your risk of suffering a stroke or heart attack. Counselling, nicotine replacement therapy and buproprion (Zyban), have all been shown to be effective in helping people quit smoking.

Why are BP-lowering drugs recommended? What is the purpose of taking them?

The doctor will hope to:

- decrease your risk of cardiovascular disease (heart attack and stroke), which can raise BP;

- decrease any risk of *coexisting* cardiovascular risk factors such as raised cholesterol, diabetes, left ventricular hypertrophy, and other conditions that raise your risk of having a cardiovascular problem; this often requires additional drug therapy, aside from BP-lowering drugs;

- improve your quality of life and encourage a healthy lifestyle.

Your risk factors, treatment preferences and social circumstances will be taken into account to match the drugs to your 'risk profile'. So treatment is chosen to ensure that any side effects of drugs are minimized.

There are several different classes of BP-lowering drugs. You will probably be given a thiazide diuretic first. Depending on other risk factors, other BP-lowering drugs can be chosen to reduce BP and minimize side effects – so called 'tailoring' of BP-lowering medication. Over two-thirds of people with raised BP require two or more different BP-lowering drugs before the ideal BP level is reached.

Follow-up

People with high BP will be registered, reviewed and recalled regularly in order to get the best out of your treatment, so you will have to be prepared to take part in an organized system of monitoring and care.

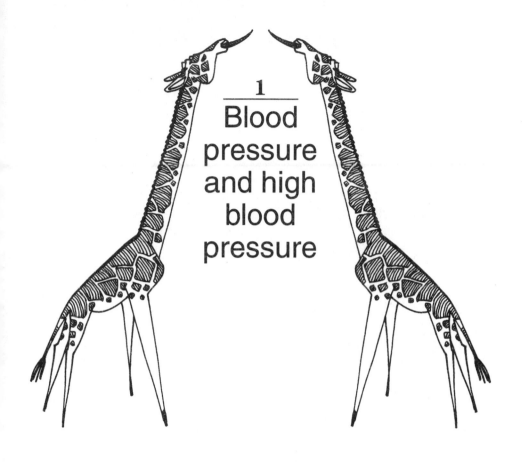

1
Blood pressure and high blood pressure

Blood pressure is needed to maintain circulation in your body so that oxygen and other nutrients can be transported to your cells. When your blood preessure is too high, it can damage the tissues and cells in your body. In this chapter the different types of high blood pressure are explained and the scale of the problem of high blood pressure in the community is outlined.

About blood pressure in general

I don't think I'd ever thought about blood being under pressure before I was told I had high blood pressure. Why should blood be under pressure?

The function of blood is to transport materials around the body, mainly to take oxygen and food substances to body cells to keep them alive and well, and to remove their waste products such as carbon dioxide. If your blood were not under some pressure, it would just stay where it is, stagnant, neither nourishing nor cleansing the cells of your body, so that within about 7 minutes first they and then you would die.

How does blood move around the body?

The circulatory system consists of two circular systems of tubes, circulation through your lungs (pulmonary circulation) and circulation through the rest of your body (systemic circulation). Blood is moved through these two systems by two pumps, the right and left sides of the heart. Although these right and left pumps beat together, the blood in each side is entirely separate, and the two pumps can, and do to some extent, function independently. Because pushing blood through your lungs is much easier than pushing it through every other part of your body, the left side of the heart is bigger, more muscular, and carries a much heavier workload than the right.

Obviously blood is under pressure at all points throughout both systems, in arteries, capillaries (the smaller vessels) and veins, otherwise it would not circulate. Pressure in capillaries is not only extremely small, but has to be kept constant, so that conditions for transfer of oxygen and nutrients into, and carbon dioxide and waste products out of, each body cell remain unchanged, despite huge differences in what the rest of your body may be doing. In fact the main reason for variability in your arterial BP is the need to keep capillary BP the same.

Obviously more pressure is needed to push blood up against gravity than to push it down. The animals that have to cope with the biggest changes in BP are therefore giraffes, whose brain capillary BP has to be kept constant whether their heads are 2 metres or so below their hearts when they drink, or 2 metres above them when they are eating leaves off the trees. For this reason, a giraffe adorns each chapter of this book, in an effort to reassure you that the text is not unreadable!

Pressure is generally much higher in arteries than in veins. When doctors talk about 'blood pressure', they normally mean arterial pressure. It is important to understand this. If you cough, sneeze, push your car out of a ditch, or strain hard sitting on the toilet, you go red in the face and you can feel your head filling up with blood. This is caused by raised BP in your veins (venous pressure), not in your arteries (arterial pressure). Many people imagine that high BP causes similar symptoms, but this is completely wrong.

Arterial pressure is highest close to the heart and diminishes as blood moves further out along the arterial tree. Arterial pressure is most easily measured in the arm just above the elbow (in the brachial artery), so this has long been the international standard way of measuring BP.

The pressure of a fluid flowing through any tube depends on four main variables:

- A   the rate at which fluid enters the tube
- B   the diameter of the tube
- C   the friction from its walls
- D   the viscosity (stickiness and elasticity) and volume of the fluid.

Likewise in your body:

- A   Your heart pumps blood into your arteries at a variable rate, depending on both what you are doing and what you are thinking.
- B   Your smaller arteries are of variable diameter, depending on tension in a spiral muscle, encircling

them in much the same way as the spiral wire in a
vacuum cleaner hose; this tension in turn depends
mainly on fast signals from the brain and slow signals
from various circulating chemicals (hormones) released
from other organs.

- C Friction along artery walls increases as they get older,
  rougher, and furred up with waxy plaques made of a
  mixture of clotted blood and cholesterol (this process
  of roughening raises BP by increasing resistance to
  blood flow, and is itself speeded up by raised pressure –
  a vicious circle).

- D Finally, both the viscosity and the volume of blood vary,
  depending mainly on salt intake, the efficiency of your
  kidneys, and the size and shape of red blood cells,
  which may be much altered by low levels of blood iron
  or high levels of blood alcohol.

**Blood pressure seems to be written down as a fraction, for
example 150/85. What do these figures represent, and
what do they mean?**

If you stick a vertical glass tube into a large human artery, blood
will rise about 9 metres (30 feet) up the tube, to the point where
the weight of the atmosphere balances the pressure supporting
the column of blood (the Reverend Stephen Hales did this in the
18th century, using a live horse). As 9–12 metre (30–40 foot) tubes
of air were inconvenient, they were replaced by tubes of mercury;
as puncturing an artery is painful, the pressure required to stop
pumping sounds from the heart became used as an indirect way
of measuring pressure inside the artery. Since about 1900, BP has
been measured in this way in millimetres of mercury (mmHg),
with the use of an 'indirect sphygmomanometer'.

If you put an ear (or, more conveniently, a stethoscope) over a
large artery in the crook of your elbow, you will hear nothing; but,
if you squeeze the artery with an inflatable cuff until it is
completely blocked above the listening point, and then very
slowly release it, you will first hear clear, regular tapping sounds,

then these will disappear. The level of pressure at which these sounds are first heard is 'systolic pressure', the pressure at which blood is first pushed out of the heart into the arteries. If you keep listening, while slowly dropping the pressure in the cuff, the tapping disappears. Then, at a pressure about 50–100 mmHg lower, you will hear regular but much softer whooshing sounds, which will also disappear after a further fall of 5–10 mmHg. The point at which these soft sounds disappear is 'diastolic pressure', the pressure of blood in the arteries between heart beats. At one time doctors disagreed about whether to define diastolic pressure as appearance or disappearance of the whooshing sound, but there is now international agreement to accept disappearance.

BP is normally recorded as systolic/diastolic, for example 105/54 mmHg (an unusually low pressure), 125/70 mmHg (an average-ish pressure), 164/95 mmHg (a high-ish pressure), 182/106 mmHg (a definitely high pressure) or 235/140 mmHg (a dangerously high pressure).

Should I know what my own figures are?

In our opinion, yes, and we think that you should know them as actual figures rather than as general statements like 'high', 'normal' or 'low'. Other doctors will ask you about your BP and, without some figures, your answers will be as meaningless to them as to you. You should also know what your overall risk is of suffering a stroke or heart attack). You should appreciate that your BP reading will vary.

How and why does BP vary so much?

Figure 1.1 shows the pattern of BP readings measured every 5 minutes throughout 24 hours in a person with a completely normal BP. Measurements were made very accurately through a polythene catheter pushed into an artery in his arm, following a local anaesthetic to ensure a painless procedure, which would not itself affect BP.

As you see, his BP varied throughout the day, with a sustained fall during sleep, a marked rise when somebody pushed a pin into

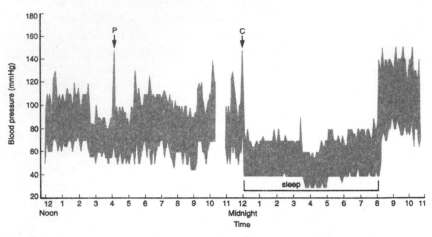

Figure 1.1 Variations in blood pressure during 24 hours in a person with normal blood pressure. Systolic pressures are shown at the top of the shaded area, and diastolic pressures at the bottom.

his skin (marked P on the chart), another when he made love (marked C), and another sustained rise during the first half of the morning. This pattern of rises and falls is typical not only of people with normal BP, but also of those with high BP.

Everyone, whether their BP is high or low, has mechanisms for distributing varying amounts of blood to different parts of the body, depending on what they are doing. For example, if you are thinking hard, your brain needs a larger blood flow than when you are asleep; after a large meal you need a much larger blood flow to your gut; and, if you are running, blood flow to all your large muscles is enormously increased.

In a normal man or woman, total blood flow at rest is about 6 litres (about 10.5 pints) a minute, with about 13% going to your brain, 24% to your gut, 21% to your large muscles, 19% to your kidneys, and 4% to your heart muscle. If you run as hard as you can, blood flow to your brain remains exactly the same, but total flow through your body as a whole rises more than four-fold to 25 litres (95 pints) a minute. Flow through your heart muscle rises four-fold, and through other large muscles ten-fold, but falls to four times less than at rest in your kidneys, and fives times less in your gut. These changes begin even if you just think about running; your body prepares for action by redistributing blood flow, and a substantial rise in BP is part of this process. In this way BP responds quickly, though usually for only a short time, to emotional states such as fear, embarrassment, anger, sexual interest, and even simple curiosity.

Between this high-pressure network of arteries conveying blood from the lungs and heart, and the low-pressure network of veins taking it back again, lies a vast mesh of microscopically small capillaries, their walls made of extremely thin cells through which molecules of oxygen, nutrients and cellular waste products can be easily exchanged. For these delicate but vital transactions to take place, pressure within the capillaries must remain constant, within very narrow limits. Given these huge shifts in blood flow between organs, this constancy can be maintained only by precise control of flow through small arteries and arterioles.

This control is mainly exerted through changes in tension in the spiral muscle surrounding the smallest arteries (arterioles), which result in big changes in arterial BP.

My BP seems to change throughout the day. Is this normal?

Figure 1.2 shows BP patterns taken from people while they are attending a hypertension hospital clinic. As you can see, there is a 'diurnal' pattern to normal BP (in other words, BP changes throughout the day). In addition, there are many other different types of patterns of high BP that vary between different people. 'White coat hypertension' will be discussed in Chapter 3 – this occurs as a response to BP measurement itself. Isolated systolic hypertension occurs more commonly in elderly people. The other patterns shown in the figure will also require BP-lowering drug treatment. Most often, detailed 24-hour readings are not necessary and the 'prognostic' significance between these different types of BP readings (whether one type of ambulatory reading is more harmful than another type of reading in terms of risk of stroke or heart attack) over a 24-hour period is not substantial.

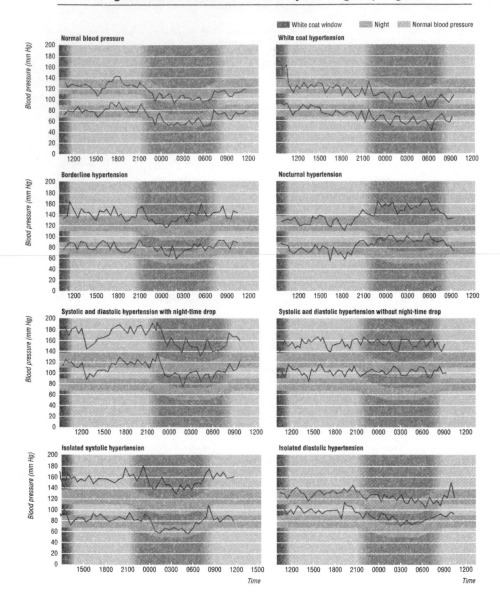

Figure 1.2 Ambulatory blood pressure patterns taken from people attending a hospital hypertension clinic.

(Charts taken from BMJ 2000 320:1131, with kind permission from the BMJ Publishing Group.)

Low blood pressure

Presumably, if there are people with high BP, then there can be also be people with low BP. Does low BP cause symptoms?

You are correct. There are people who have low BP. Most people have no symptoms from their low BP. However, if BP in your neck arteries is not high enough to supply the oxygen and glucose needed to support the full function of your brain cells, you lose consciousness – that is, you faint. In teenagers (particularly girls) this happens easily and often, because their BP is generally very low (systolic pressures under 100 mmHg are common), and often less stable than in mature adults. The same thing will happen if your BP is brought down too low by overtreatment.

There is no evidence that 'low BP' justifies prescription of drugs such as non-steroidal anti-inflammatory drugs (NSAIDs) to raise BP, although this is quite commonly done in Germany. In the UK there has been a professional consensus against this practice.

High blood pressure

What is high blood pressure?

I have heard my doctor use the word 'hypertension'. Is this the same as high BP?

Yes, there is no difference: these words are used interchangeably by doctors, but have the same meaning.

I always thought that 'hypertension' implied a main cause (stress or tension) and therefore conveys more meaning than 'high BP'. Is it not therefore a better name?

No. The word 'hypertension' comes from translating the French *tension arterielle*. This originally referred not to psychological or physical tension in the mind, but to tension (stretching) of artery walls. Tension in the mind is one possible cause of high BP in some people, but is certainly not the main cause in everybody.

My husband has high BP, but he seems to be just as well as everyone else in our family. So is high BP really an illness?

With the exception of 'malignant' high BP (there is a question about this in the *Types of high blood pressure* section later in this chapter), high BP is not an illness that you either do or do not have. Rather it is a risk marker for other illnesses that you would wish to avoid. These include stroke, heart attacks, kidney problems and other problems affecting the circulatory system. Most people (like your husband) have high BP but do not have any symptoms. However, not having symptoms does not imply that he is not at risk of having any of the potential harmful consequences of having high BP. His risk of suffering complications can be reduced by non-drug or drug treatment and he also will need to address other risk factors, for example smoking, that increase his overall risk.

Is there a dividing line between normal and high BP?

Research has shown that at every level of BP, higher BP means a higher risk of stroke, heart attacks and other circulatory problems – all these are considered as 'cardiovascular' risks. So there is no conventional level below which BP is 'normal'. Risk of any of these problems is related specifically to your level of BP. Added to your level of BP are other important contributory factors to your overall level of risk of stroke, heart disease and other cardiovascular problems. These include your age, sex, cholesterol level, smoking status, height and weight (as reflected in your body mass index [BMI] – see Chapter 4). It is for this reason that your overall risk of cardiovascular illness will be estimated.

Assuming that you have had enough careful measurements to measure your average BP correctly, the truth is that 'normal' BP becomes high at the point where the advantages of being supervised by your doctor (and probably eventual medication) outweigh the disadvantages. This will also depend on your overall level of cardiovascular risk and on whether you are prepared to take BP-lowering drugs or not.

I haven't had any symptoms despite my BP being high. Why does it need to be treated?

The only reason anyone needs treatment for high BP is to prevent its likely consequences – what we call 'cardiovascular risk'. Many serious sorts of organ damage are eventually caused by high BP, including all forms of stroke, coronary heart attacks, heart failure, retinal damage in your eyes, obstruction of blood flow in leg arteries, stretching ('aneurysm') of the aorta with consequent high risk of bursting ('rupture') of the aorta, and damage to the kidneys leading eventually to kidney ('renal') failure.

All these problems happen more often in people with uncontrolled high BP, and the higher the pressure is, the more likely they are to occur. After a few years of treatment, these risks become roughly proportional to the level of BP after treatment, not to the level of BP before treatment – so careful treatment works.

High BP is not the only cause of these kinds of organ damage, so reducing BP cannot wholly prevent them. Smoking is another very important cause of all of them, and so are high blood cholesterol levels and diabetes, which are often associated with being overweight and doing insufficient regular exercise. Prevention is more effective if these factors are addressed.

Types of high blood pressure

Are there different kinds of high BP?

Indeed there are, and probably more than we know of at the present time.

High BP was traditionally classified into two main groups:

- rare cases for which causes were known ('secondary hypertension' – in other words, where high BP is secondary to some other condition), and

- common cases where no cause was known ('essential hypertension'). 'Essential' did not mean that the high BP was necessary, but that it was 'of the essence': in other words, you had it because you had it, for reasons unknown. This word is now beginning to give way to the more commonsense terms of 'primary hypertension', or 'primary high BP'.

Secondary high BP is mostly caused by various sorts of kidney disease, or occasionally by malformations of the aorta ('coarctation'), overproduction of some BP-raising hormones by tumours of the pituitary gland, adrenal glands or kidneys, or by disorders involving compression of the brain or brain stem. These 'classical' secondary causes altogether used to account for less than 1% of all treated cases of high BP. If we exclude high BP caused by the oral contraceptive pill, this remains true today.

As 'essential' high BP was by definition of unknown cause, the category has inevitably become more and more unreal, as more interacting causes are found. We now have the situation that many important causes are known, which, if dealt with early, can lead to a fall in BP, but these have not yet been reclassified as 'secondary hypertension'. Examples are being overweight and drinking too much alcohol in young men, mostly those with a family history of high BP and therefore genetically susceptible to these causes. As more real causes are discovered, even primary hypertension will eventually have to be recognized as a diverse group.

If doctors know all this, then why do they still use the terms like 'essential hypertension' or 'primary high BP'?

The category remains useful because, although causes are diverse, consequences of uncontrolled high BP, and methods of controlling it, are not. Whatever the cause of high BP, risks of stroke, heart failure, coronary disease and various other sorts of organ damage are increased. Perhaps even more importantly, no convincing or consistent evidence has yet been found that different causes would benefit much from different medication.

In practice, the aim of treatment is usually not to find causes and treat them, but to find medication that works and is well tolerated, and then to keep on prescribing it. In some ways this is a realistic acceptance of the limitations of current medical knowledge, but this attitude also leads to very widespread neglect of other measures (such as weight reduction and alcohol restriction, which can be equally effective, particularly in young people), and great wealth for pharmaceutical companies.

I heard the words 'malignant hypertension' mentioned in the papers recently? Does it have anything to do with cancer?

No, despite the name, it has nothing to do with cancer, but it is the most serious form of high BP and can cause immense damage (and even death) in a very short time.

Malignant high BP is a medical emergency. If it is not recognized and treated urgently, irreversible damage of the kidney, retina and brain are likely in a very short time – delays before starting treatment should be measured in hours rather than days. Before effective treatment of high BP became available in the 1950s, death rates from malignant high BP were normally 100% within 2 years, mostly from heart failure, kidney failure or massive stroke. Many people became blind or paralysed long before this.

As more and more people with high BP are picked up early by routine measurements of BP, it is becoming rare. Malignant high BP does not occur unless either very high BP has persisted for a long time, usually several years, or BP rises very fast indeed, with no time for artery walls to thicken and resist this pressure.

Although many people with malignant high BP get severe headache, others may have severe kidney damage and very high pressures without any symptoms at all. Anyone with a severe headache should have their BP measured immediately, although high BP is rarely the cause. Another common early symptom is blurred vision or patchy loss of vision starting in one eye. Anyone with a diastolic pressure over 120 mmHg might have malignant high BP, so tests will include a urine test for protein and a retinal examination with an ophthalmoscope, either in a dark room or after putting drops into the eyes to dilate the pupils. Today, if malignant high BP is found, you would normally be sent into hospital urgently, and BP will brought down gradually over the next 2–3 days. Subsequent treatment is usually the same as for all other cases of high BP, but will be maintained for the rest of your life.

So what exactly is happening in malignant high BP?

If BP remains very high for weeks, months or years, with a sustained diastolic pressure of at least 120 mmHg (usually much more), the walls of the smallest arteries (arterioles) begin to crumble. Blood then leaks out of them, interrupting the supply of arterial blood wherever they happen to be. This usually begins in the kidney, where damage leads to release of hormones, which push BP up even higher, thus setting up a vicious circle of acceleration, in which already very high BP pushes itself higher still.

The next site of arteriolar damage is usually the retina, causing leaks of blood ('retinal haemorrhages') and leaks of plasma ('retinal exudates'). Finally, there is arteriolar damage to the brain, causing first swelling of the head of the optic nerve, then fits, and finally small strokes, unless the whole sequence is interrupted by heart failure.

The scale of the problem

How many people have high BP?

High BP is the commonest major disorder seen and tackled by doctors. BP high enough to require some kind of medical treatment and continuing supervision affects between 10 and 30% of the adult population, depending on age, and ethnic or social background. This compares with 2–8% of the adult population for diabetes, a disorder of comparable significance for health.

Is it a growing or diminishing problem?

There is no evidence that average BP in the general population has risen over the 70 or so years over which measurements are available. There is some evidence from the USA that it may have diminished, and that this reduction is due to the increasing use of BP-lowering drugs over the last 30 years. Whatever definition of high BP is used (and this has varied a good deal, since all definitions are arbitrary), the proportion of people with high BP is directly related to average pressure throughout the population.

Standardized and accurate BP measurements for large representative populations have been available in the UK, Scandinavia and the USA only since the 1950s, and more recently for other countries. There is some evidence from countries whose national diet has shifted from very high to much lower sodium intakes, notably Japan, Portugal and Belgium, that average BP in the general population has fallen, probably for this reason. These reductions in sodium intake reflect shifts in methods of food preservation from salting, smoking and pickling, to refrigeration and rapid transport of fresh food. As these changes have occurred in all economically developed societies, BP has probably fallen everywhere, compared with average levels in the 19th century.

This view is supported by trends in death rates from stroke, which are known to depend more on average BP than on any other factor. In every country that collects complete and reliable data on deaths by medically certified cause, stroke rates have been falling, probably since the 1920s, certainly since the 1950s.

Are you more likely to get high BP if you're rich rather than if you're poor?

No, it's the other way around. Research has shown higher average BPs in poorer people. Although these BP differences in different social classes are not large, there are also differences in other risk factors for heart disease. These differences translate into differences in rates of stroke and heart disease according to different social class.

Are there differences in BP between races, or between different sorts of societies?

High BP does not seem to exist in the few uncontaminated primitive societies that still exist, for example South American rainforest Indians on the upper Amazon, and Papua–New Guinea Highlanders. In the rest of the economically undeveloped countries, high BP is a much more serious problem than in developed economies, with very high stroke rates, particularly in rural areas, and corresponding burdens of care for these populations. In the economically less developed parts of southern and central Europe, death rates from stroke are still more than twice as great as death rates from coronary heart disease, whereas in developed European economies death rates from coronary disease are about three times as great as those from stroke.

High BP is a serious problem in the African–Caribbean black population, occurring in up to 40% of adults of this ethnic background. Amongst this group, high BP tends to be more severe and is associated with a higher risk of complications, particularly heart and kidney problems. British South Asians (from the Indian sub-continent) also have a risk of developing high BP. They are also more likely to suffer from diabetes, which acts in tandem with their high BP to increase the risk of heart attacks and strokes substantially. Well-fed people from the Indian subcontinent have very high rates for diabetes, affecting up to 12% of the middle-aged population in some immigrant communities in the UK, compared with 2–4% for ethnic Europeans. As diabetes is itself a major risk factor for stroke, populations of Indian descent have much larger

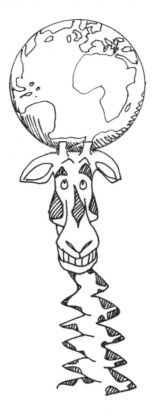

health problems related to BP control. A multiple approach, including stopping smoking, and taking cholesterol-lowering drugs and aspirin is often recommended, in order to reduce overall risk of stroke and heart attack.

It seems impossible these days to talk about anything to do with people's health without talking about money incurred by the NHS – so what are the economics of treating high BP?

This depends first on how much treatment is rational, i.e. there is good evidence that it is preventing stroke and other problems of uncontrolled high BP, and how much treatment is driven by other incentives and pressures: in private practice, these include fees;

in competitive NHS practice, they include satisfying the expectations of people (real or assumed), and for almost everyone they include pressure from the pharmaceutical industry (which, like any other industry, wishes to increase its sales and profits). Secondly, it depends on whether we see benefits in terms of health gains for people or cash relief for taxpayers.

In the UK, roughly one-fifth of the people with high BP who would benefit from treatment are not identified, one-fifth of those with known high BP are not having treatment, and half of those treated do not have their BP properly controlled. This failure to deliver care is socially distributed: those in the greatest need in the poorest sections of society often get the least care.

It is most likely that the greatest gain from the least investment would be not to look for more undiscovered and untreated people with high BP, but to reorganize the care of those already known and treated. General practices need to organize follow-up clinics so that they have lists of people who need to attend, check whether they have actually done so, and if not, ask themselves why they haven't. Research in both the USA and UK has shown that organized review and re-call clinics in the community are highly effective in helping people with high BP reach their 'goal' of reducing their BP.

A more recent change is that management of high BP is now seen in the context of overall risk of having a stroke, heart attack etc. GPs are now being encouraged to treat high BP by dealing with other major risk factors for stroke and coronary heart disease, such as lowering cholesterol and stopping smoking.

2
Symptoms, causes and diagnosis

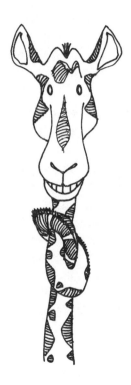

High blood pressure, as will be discussed later in this chapter, is a risk factor for heart disease and stroke. Having high blood pressure generally causes no symptoms for most people. It is only in the very rare situation of 'malignant' high blood pressure that symptoms may occur, usually in the form of headaches.

Symptoms

Do people with high BP feel any different from people with normal BP?

Usually no. By itself, before it has caused organ damage, high BP causes no symptoms at all. Symptoms may not be noticeable even after organ damage has started. Even very high pressures, very dangerous and already causing serious kidney damage, may sometimes be present for several months before they cause any symptoms. The only way to know if you have high BP (and how high it is) is to have it measured with a sphygmomanometer. There is more information about this in Chapter 3.

I have suffered from headaches and breathlessness lately – do you think these are caused by my high BP?

When BP reaches about 180/120 mmHg, some symptoms can occur: chiefly headache and breathlessness on slight exertion, such as going upstairs. Of course, both these symptoms are common anyway, but they happen more often in people with high BP, and increasingly so as BP rises. Some of these headaches can be a warning of early damage to arteries in the brain or retina, requiring urgent control of BP to prevent serious complications.

Higher levels of BP also often occur with other factors that increase the likelihood of breathlessness, for example being overweight. So it may be difficult to attribute symptoms to a single cause. Breathlessness in people with high BP is usually simply a result of being overweight but, if your BP has either risen out of control or unaccountably started to fall without any change in your medication, breathlessness may be the main symptom of early heart failure.

As lots of people get headaches from anxiety, tension, or minor virus infections, such innocent headaches are equally common in people with high BP, but a careful doctor will always check BP first, before dismissing associated headaches as insignificant; they could occasionally signal sudden dangerous loss of control in your BP. Do visit your doctor to make sure that your BP is being adequately controlled.

I would have thought that increased BP would sometimes cause bleeding. Isn't this so?

Risk of bleeding from arteries into the brain (causing stroke) or into the retina (the back of the eye, causing patchy loss of vision if the bleed is large) is increased by high BP, particularly in people over 50, and is one of the main reasons why high BP needs treatment.

Nosebleeds and small bleeds into the white of the eye ('subconjunctival haemorrhages') can occur in people with high BP, although both are common in people with normal BP and need not necessarily be a cause for alarm. Subconjunctival haemorrhage sounds alarming, but the word 'haemorrhage' is simply a posh word for bleeding of any extent, large or small. Subconjunctival haemorrhages appear, often after coughing, sneezing or straining on the toilet, and disappear slowly over the next 6 weeks. They are completely harmless and have nothing to do with retinal haemorrhages.

Heavy periods and other menopausal symptoms, including palpitations, sweats and the sensation with or without the appearance of flushing, all occur commonly in women with high BP, simply because high BP is common at this age. None of these symptoms is caused by high BP, or cured by lowering it.

Since I was told I had high BP, I've had awful palpitations. Is this one of the symptoms, and why didn't I notice it before?

Palpitations (feeling or hearing your own heart beating fast), tension headaches and overbreathing are common in people who are anxious or frightened. If they have these symptoms already, and are then found to have high BP, this may confirm their fears and reinforce the symptoms. People without such symptoms, after they have been told that they have high BP, often get palpitations for the first time, not because of high BP, but because of fear of high BP. With sufficient explanation of what this diagnosis actually means, symptoms usually disappear, although not always immediately.

Although I'm only 35, my doctor says I have unusually high BP. I've noticed that my heart often seems to miss a beat and, if I count my pulse, it's often irregular. Has this got something to do with high BP?

Almost certainly not. There are two common causes of an irregular pulse in young adults such as yourself.

- If you take long, deep breaths, you may find that your wrist pulse slows down as you breathe in, and speeds up as you breathe out. This is not a sign of disease, but of youth. It is caused by a link between the nerves controlling breathing movements of the diaphragm and the point of origin of heartbeats, the 'atrial sinus'; it is therefore called 'sinus arrhythmia'. Older people lose this link, but some still have it well into their 50s.

- The second common cause, at all ages, is extra heart beats ('extrasystoles'). These are smaller, relatively ineffective heartbeats, too small to reach the wrist, but they cause an apparent delay before the next beat that is big enough to feel. They are completely normal and harmless, and always disappear if you start any vigorous activity.

Irregular heartbeats in older people may be more complicated, and be due to irregular movement of the upper chambers of the heart ('atrial fibrillation'). They can occur when BP is poorly controlled, and need to be confirmed by an electrocardiograph (ECG), an electronic tracing of the heart. As atrial fibrillation is a strong risk factor for suffering a stroke, treatment with blood-thinning drugs (usually warfarin or aspirin) is needed. There is more information about this condition in Chapter 6.

Causes

Does anybody know what really causes high BP?

There is still a lot of uncertainty about the causes of high BP. For the vast majority of people, over 95%, an underlying cause is not found. These are the individuals who have 'essential' hypertension (see Chapter 1). It is likely that several interrelated factors contribute to high BP in most people. The chief suspects include:

- an overactive hormone system that relates to the kidney (the 'renin–angiotensin system');

- an overactive autonomic nervous system (the part of the nervous system that is responsible for our unconscious nervous responses);

- a fault in the cells of the smaller blood vessels that produce substances leading to blood vessel narrowing and increased BP ('endothelial cell dysfunction');

- genetic predisposition (when you have inherited a tendency to high BP);

- factors occurring at birth, particularly birth weight, possibly reflecting undernourishment in the fetus, which 'programme' our body to develop high BP in later life.

I have always thought that physical or psychological stress and tension raises BP. Is that right?

Yes, and this is where confusion arises. Both real and imagined stress cause a large rise in BP, lasting minutes or even hours. Such rises are normal and occur in everyone. They are brief additions to their usual average pressure, high or low. As a cause of eventual organ damage, however, 'high BP' refers not to these peaks, but to the steady average level over weeks, months or years, to which BP returns when stress is removed.

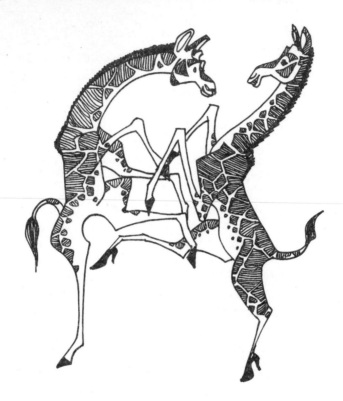

My father had high blood pressure. Is high BP inherited?

Although genetic factors have been linked to the development of essential hypertension, multiple genes are most likely to contribute to the development of the disorder in a particular individual. Therefore, in any one individual, high BP is hardly ever simply an inherited disease like muscular dystrophy, Huntington's disease or haemophilia. A rare exception is polycystic disease of the kidney, mostly determined by a single 'dominant' gene, and therefore occurring in 50% of offspring of a single affected parent.

In terms of inheritance, high BP is about twice as common in people who have one or two hypertensive parents. When populations are studied, at least a third of the variance in BP within large populations can be predicted from knowledge of BP in parents and brothers and sisters.

In all other cases, BP depends on interaction between many different inherited factors, many of which operate only if certain environmental conditions exist. The most important of these are probably birth weight, adolescent and early adult growth, salt and alcohol intake.

If I have high BP myself, are my children more likely to develop high BP? If so, is there anything I can do about it?

Children of parents with high BP are more likely to develop high BP themselves. In terms of prevention, the general recommendations of taking regular exercise, maintaining a healthy diet and avoiding becoming overweight are particularly relevant. However, there are no unique or different recommendations for individuals with a family history of high BP than there are for those without such a history.

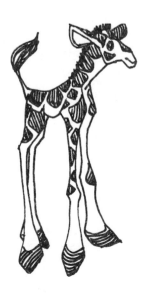

I take quite a few drugs altogether. Would any of the drugs I am taking cause high BP?

Yes. Four groups of medicines or drugs might cause high blood pressure: home remedies bought across the counter at the chemist, herbal medicines, drugs of addiction and abuse, and prescribed medication.

- **Home remedies bought over the counter.** Many different preparations available for shrinking up the air passages in your nose during colds, hay fever ('allergic rhinitis') or 'chronic catarrh' (usually unrecognized hay fever) can raise BP, because they contain chemicals closely related to naturally occurring chemicals in the body that influence BP. If you are using any kind of nasal decongestant, make sure you mention this to anyone who may be measuring your BP. Despite their popularity, nasal decongestants containing these drugs (sympathomimetic amines) only work for a short time, and cause rebound swelling as soon as they are stopped. This leads many people to go on using them for days, months or even years on end, in which case they develop severe chronic obstruction in the nose, and catarrh, caused by the very drug that they are using to treat it. This dependence is reinforced by the fact that these drugs tend to wake people up and give them a bit of a lift, in the same way as dexamphetamine (Dexedrine, 'speed') does, so that (often unconsciously) they become addicted to them. The moral is, don't use them unless you have to, and never use them for more than a couple of hours. Traditional remedies such as menthol and eucalyptus are safer and just as effective, but check with your chemist that they don't contain amine supplements.

- **Drugs of addiction and abuse.** Dexamphetamine and its more potent and even more dangerous relation 'Ecstasy', causes a high mood, wakefulness, indifference to food, and very high BP. Both drugs can cause hallucinations, which may be dangerous if people drive, and, combined with vigorous activity at high room temperature, 'Ecstasy' may raise BP high enough to cause death from acute heart failure. Cocaine may also cause prolonged rises in BP, and so, of course, may alcohol.

- **Herbal medicines.** Herbal remedies that can cause high BP or interact with BP-lowering medication may make BP-lowering drugs less effective. If you suffer from atrial fibrillation (see Chapter 6) and take blood-thinning medication (warfarin or aspirin), herbal products are known to interact and prolong the action of blood-thinning medication. Before you take any herbal remedy, it is always better to discuss with a pharmacist whether it is likely to have any unwanted side effects.

- **Prescribed medication.** Prescribed drugs include non-steroidal anti-inflammatory drugs (NSAIDs), drugs derived from liquorice, which were at one time used commonly to treat gastric ulcer but are now rarely prescribed, and some steroid hormones. NSAIDs are commonly used for joint pain. They can increase BP by 5–6 mmHg diastolic pressure, about the same amount as many BP-lowering drugs bring it down. Many of these are now available from chemists over the counter, of which the most widely consumed is ibuprofen (Brufen). Because of this effect, it is important that you remind your doctor or pharmacist that you have high BP if you ever need painkillers, as they will be able to suggest more suitable alternatives for you.

  Corticosteroid hormones include cortisone, hydro-cortisone, prednisone, prednisolone, and adrenocortico-trophic hormone (ACTH). All of them raise BP by causing sodium and water retention and thus increasing blood volume, if given in high dosage. This normally happens only if steroids are taken into the body as tablets or injections, but heavy use of some strong steroid ointments may penetrate sufficiently through the skin to have the same effect. These big doses should never be used other than for serious, usually life-threatening disease, which will be treated by hospital specialists. The only conditions in which steroid treatment is at all likely to interfere with management of high BP are severe asthma and rheumatoid arthritis. These are discussed in Chapter 6.

I'm 30, I don't smoke and, although I do enjoy an occasional glass of wine, I'm not a heavy drinker – but I've got high BP, which I'd always thought only affected people who were much older than me. Are the causes of high BP in people of my age just the same as for people who are middle-aged or older?

Generally yes, bearing in mind that we don't know most of the causes of much of the high BP in middle-aged and elderly people. The main difference is that, in younger adults like you, there are other rare secondary causes (usually relating to the kidney or adrenal glands). Younger people who developed high BP used to be referred to hospital, but this situation has now changed and investigation of high BP can be carried out by your doctor, usually by means of checking your urine for protein and performing simple blood tests.

Is getting older or just being old in itself a cause of high BP? In other words, is high BP normal in old age?

Blood pressure, particularly systolic BP, rises with age. It is now accepted that, although high BP in the elderly is common, it should not be accepted as normal. In fact the consequences of high BP, particularly stroke and heart attacks, are far more common in the elderly. Clinical trials of BP-lowering drugs have shown that treatment of elderly people with high BP is highly effective and cost effective. The consequence is that elderly people are now commonly treated for high BP, with up to one-fifth of people aged over 65 in the UK taking BP-lowering drugs.

Diagnosis

How do doctors diagnose high BP?

Measuring your BP is by far the most important routine test before a diagnosis can be made. It is very important that you have repeated measurements of your BP over time, so as to make sure that your average reading is estimated accurately. At a minimum, three readings should be taken on four or more separate occasions. For all but very severe cases of high BP, decisions about treatment are much better after 2 weeks or so of twice-daily home readings. As BP measurement is so important, it is covered as a separate topic in the next chapter.

I am going for my repeat BP test next week as my first one was high. What questions will I be asked?

Any doctor or nurse who is meeting you to find out why you have high BP will ask questions, examine you and order investigations in a structured manner. The following list is an outline of what you might expect to be asked:

- Was the BP measurement different from or the same as your normal BP?
- Did this measurement worry you?
- Did you hurry to your appointment?
- Was it very cold outside?
- Had you a full bladder?
- Was there any other reason why any kind of discomfort or anxiety might have pushed up your BP?

Doctors or nurses measuring BP are all taught to look for reasons of this sort for unexpectedly high values, but many are too rushed themselves to do so. A rapid pulse often gives a clue to anxiety or vigorous exercise within the previous 10–15 minutes.

You will then be asked questions about yourself, your past medical and family history and other associated risks that you might have that are associated with high BP. In more detail the following points should be covered:

- A note of your current age and sex.

- A review of some important symptoms that you might have. These are important when assessing whether you have ever suffered any complications from having high BP. Questions will include any recent symptoms of: chest pain; shortness of breath; dizziness episodes; blurred vision; slurred speech; memory loss; leg pain.

- Your past medical history, which might include heart attack ('myocardial infarct'); angina; stroke; transient ischaemic attack (TIA – a mini-stroke where symptoms of weakness resolve entirely within 24 hours); memory loss; left ventricular hypertrophy (thickening of the heart vessel wall); heart failure; heart operations including coronary angioplasty or bypass surgery; diabetes, kidney disease (a broad term for a variety of different conditions that result in reduced kidney function; in some situations, where kidney function reduces progressively over time, 'end-stage' kidney failure occurs where the kidney's excretory function breaks down and you would require dialysis), and coarctation of the aorta (narrowing of the main blood vessel leading from the heart).

- Whether anybody in your family had an early stroke or a heart atack or diabetes.

- Your family history of high BP. People without any family history of high BP are more likely to have a rare, surgically treatable cause of high BP, such as a kidney disorder or coarctation of the aorta.

- Whether you smoke, drink excessively and what your diet is like.

- What drugs you are taking, specifically those that are associated with having high BP: corticosteroids; non-steroidal anti-inflammatory drugs (NSAIDs); amphetamines (appetite suppressants); caffeine intake, sympathomimetics (found in nasal decongestants or bronchodilators); oral contraceptives; sodium-containing medications (antacids).

You will then be examined and the following tests should be done:

- Your BP levels will be measured – the way in which this is done and how often it is done is critical to whether you are classified as having high BP or not. Chapter 3 covers BP measurement in more detail.

- Your height and weight will be measured, which will allow the doctor or nurse to calculate your body mass index (see Chapter 4).

- You should be examined for absent or suspiciously reduced pulses over the femoral arteries, felt in your groin creases. This is the classical sign of coarctation of the aorta, rare but easily detected, for which there is very effective surgical treatment.

- "End organ' damage (damage caused to the eyes, heart, circulation and kidney owing to prolonged high blood pressure) will be assessed. This includes an eye examination, looking for fundal haemorrhages or exudates; an examination of your heart, looking for evidence of heart failure or left ventricular hypertrophy.

- Your abdomen will be examined so that any swelling of your aorta (main artery in your body) can be excluded.

Remember that 'classical' causes of secondary high BP are all rare, accounting for less than 1% of all cases of treated high BP. In practice they are usually searched for in two stages: before treatment begins and if treatment unaccountably fails.

Will the doctor do some tests straightaway?

All people should have the following tests done as early as possible:

- **Urine test:** to check for protein and sugar in the urine. Leakage of protein may indicate that the kidneys have been damaged from high BP and you will need more detailed assessment of your kidney function. Testing for sugar is a relatively straightforward way of checking for diabetes. Similarly, if sugar is present, then blood tests will be needed to confirm or rule out diabetes.

- **Blood tests:** to measure urea, electrolytes and creatinine levels; total cholesterol/HDL cholesterol.

- **X-rays and ECGs:** Routine chest X-rays and X-rays of the kidney ('pyelography') are not necessary or useful for routine initial assessment. Electrocardiograms (ECGs) give much less information about heart function than most people think. They require careful evaluation, and interpretation is full of pitfalls. However, interpretation of any future chest pain is far easier if a baseline ECG is available. One single ECG trace is therefore a useful investigation for everyone, before starting treatment. *After* onset of suspicious chest pains, an ECG is essential.

I have been diagnosed with high BP. What tests and investigations will be done to find out why I have this?

Before starting treatment, everybody should be tested for possible kidney damage by simple urine tests for protein, bacteria and glucose, and by measuring blood urea and creatinine levels. These may indicate a cause for your high BP in your kidneys; this accounts for more than half of all cases of classical secondary high BP. At the same time a number of other routine blood tests are usually requested, including three that often give clues to high alcohol intake (raised mean corpuscular volume, gamma-glutamyl transferase and triglyceride levels), and one that indicates rare adrenal tumours that raise BP (reduced blood potassium).

Routine chest X-rays and special X-rays of the kidney ('pyelography') were thought at one time to be essential before starting treatment. Many trials have since confirmed that these are not efficient ways of looking for secondary high BP at this stage, unless there are other definite indications of heart failure, lung or kidney disease.

If, after several months of treatment, your BP is not controlled or, if after several years of good control, your BP becomes uncontrollable despite continued treatment, a secondary cause will be sought, starting with investigations to see whether one of your kidney arteries has been blocked by a clot. Some very rare causes, such as the adrenal tumour phaeochromocytoma, are extremely difficult to find.

Will my visit to the clinic be the only one I have to attend? How many readings and visits are needed before high BP is diagnosed?

There is no universally accepted number of visits that are necessary to establish a diagnosis of high BP. However, all national guidelines recommend several visits and several readings before high BP is diagnosed. Clinical trials that established the benefits of BP-lowering treatments generally used two or three BP readings on three or more clinic visits to establish the diagnosis.

I am aged 74 and have recently been told that I have high BP. During the initial consultation my doctor showed me a chart and told me that my cardiovascular risk was high. What does all this mean?

Guidelines now state that high BP should not be seen and treated on its own without also taking into account your risk of suffering a stroke or heart attack). Factors such as age, gender, history of diabetes, smoking status, serum cholesterol, family history and past history of possible strokes and heart attacks, all contribute

to your level of cardiovascular risk. Charts that rank people into levels of such risk have now been published and can be found on the National Heart Foundation of New Zealand's website:
    www.nzgg.org.nz/library/gl_complete/bloodpressure/table1.cfm,
and many general practitioners use these charts. Examples of these are included in Appendix 2.

A consequence of taking this type of approach is that treatment recommendations are likely to include non-drug solutions, such as taking more exercise or stopping smoking. It also means that different types of drug treatments can also be recommended, such as cholesterol-lowering drugs, BP-lowering drugs and drugs that prevent clotting (aspirin).

Some pointers as to your risk, such as age and gender, are not possible to change. Getting older is associated with an increasing risk of suffering a heart attack or stroke. Your decision of whether to start or defer treatment is very much up to you. Discussion with your doctor and nurse about taking BP-lowering drugs should be in the light of your overall risk, whether you wish to try non-drug treatments initially, and whether you are happy to take BP-lowering drugs (putting you at risk of suffering side effects) to lower your initial risk of stroke or heart attack. Some people find it helpful to consider their actual level of risk and their risk compared with an average person of their age and sex.

How do I decide to start treatment or not, based on my absolute risk of suffering a heart attack or stroke?

Absolute risk profiles and risk-based guidelines do not by themselves solve the problem of setting treatment starting points ('thresholds'). Blood pressure treatment guidelines often specify different treatment thresholds for starting BP-lowering drugs, and it is well known that people seeking help and health professionals differ in the threshold that they would choose themselves for starting to take BP-lowering drugs.

As there is a direct, linear relationship between systolic and diastolic BP and the risk of future heart attack or stroke (the higher your BP, the greater your risk), it is not surprising that there is no strong agreement as to which BP or absolute risk threshold should be chosen when deciding on BP-lowering treatment. For this reason, you should discuss with your doctor what level of absolute risk you think is acceptable before starting BP-lowering drugs. Some people find it helpful to consider their risk in the context of their absolute risk compared with somebody of the same age and sex.

If all this seems confusing, there are now several charts, CD-ROMs and websites that help you to weigh up the risks and benefits of BP-lowering drugs. You need to balance up the future potential benefit of starting BP-lowering drugs weighed against possible side effects and inconvenience of taking long-term treatment. Your doctor will also want to weigh up costs. A list of these sites and programmes is provided in Appendix 2.

Aside from these risk charts, are there any other ways to estimate my cardiovascular risk?

Risk estimation can now be undertaken on the internet using information derived from trials of BP-lowering drugs therapy (see Appendix 3 for some website details). These websites often contain information about drug and non-drug treatment of high BP.

Research has shown that people with high BP often disagree with BP guidelines and health professionals over the level of risk that they are prepared to accept as either safe or hazardous. You should view your risk assessment and BP level as the starting point for discussing the risks and benefits of BP treatment with your doctor or practice nurse. Though it can be confusing and intimidating at first, your own preferences about taking medication and about the consequences of high BP, particularly how you feel about avoiding a stroke or a heart attack, are the most important factors when you are trying to decide whether or not you wish to start taking BP medication.

3
Measuring blood pressure

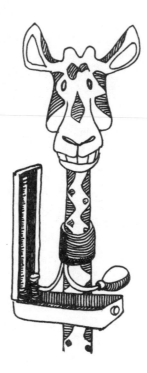

The initial starting point when high blood pressure is being assessed is for the doctor or nurse to ensure that an accurate and reliable reading is obtained. BP measurement is an area where technology is changing all the time. With the advent of electronic monitors it is now possible for you to measure your own blood pressure. The following chapter aims to give you an overview of the issues that relate to accurate and reliable blood pressure measurement.

Types of BP measuring devices

I have been called in for a BP reading. How will this be done?

Blood pressure can be measured in several ways, by means of an electronic, mercury or aneroid sphygmomanometer. 'Sphygmo-manometer' is the technical term for an instrument used to measure BP (a manometer is an instrument for measuring the pressure of fluids; *sphygmos* is the Greek word for pulse). These instruments could equally well just be called 'BP monitors' but sphygmomanometer was the name chosen when they first came into use in the late 19th century and is still used today.

The sphygmomanometer in everyday use in doctors' surgeries consists of a device for measuring BP connected to an inflatable cuff, which is wrapped around the upper arm. The differences between the three types of instrument relate to the pressure-measuring devices they use.

How does the mercury sphygmomanometer work?

The inflation/deflation mechanism is connected by rubber tubing to a bladder which envelops the arm. The cuff is inflated by squeezing a bulb by hand and deflation by means of a release valve. The pump and control valve are connected to the inflatable bladder and hence to the sphygmomanometer by rubber tubing. The doctor or nurse listens to the artery wall with a stethoscope, detecting sounds produced as blood passes through as the bladder deflates. The corresponding mercury level is then read off; this reading corresponds to the systolic BP. When these sounds disappear, the reading corresponds to the diastolic BP.

What is the best sphygmomanometer for measuring BP?

The gold standard for BP measurement is the mercury sphygmo-manometer (Figure 3.1). This instrument has been used in all the clinical trials that have assessed the effectiveness of drug treatment as described. However, mercury is now being phased

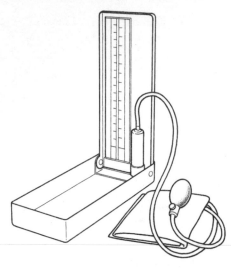

Figure 3.1 Mercury sphygmomanometer.

out in several European Union countries and has been totally replaced in Sweden and the Netherlands. Unfortunately, in some European countries, including the UK and Ireland, the move to ban mercury in hospitals and clinics has not been received with enthusiasm, as there are no alternative accurate measuring devices in common use. There are many electronic sphygmomanometers, but many of these devices are frequently inaccurate and unreliable. The British Hypertension Society has a website and this gives details of the accuracy of newer electronic sphygmomanometers against the 'gold standard' of a mercury sphygmomanometer. Prior to purchasing an electronic device, it is well to ensure that it has been validated by the British Hypertension Society. Links to the website are provided in Appendix 2.

What differences are there between the gold standard device and the other types, and why aren't they used so much?

- **Aneroid sphygmomanometers** (Figure 3.2). These devices balance BP against pressure in a thin metal capsule

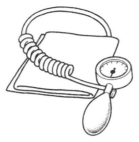

Figure 3.2 Aneroid sphygmomanometer.

containing air ('aneroid' comes from the Greek, and means 'without using fluids'). Aneroid sphygmomanometers register BP through a bellows and lever system, which is mechanically more complex and intricate than the mercury reservoir and column. The problem with the aneroid sphygmomanometer is that it frequently becomes inaccurate over time. The reason for this is that the jolts of everyday use affects the instruments. Checks have shown that a third or more of aneroid sphygmomanometers may be out by up to 4 mmHg or more when calibrated against a mercury sphygmomanometer. Up to 10% may be 10 mmHg or more out. For these reasons aneroid sphygmomanometers are no longer recommended for clinical use.

- **Electronic sphygmomanometers** (Figure 3.3). Automated sphygmomanometers can eliminate several important sources of error and are easy to use, particularly by people measuring their own BP at home. Unfortunately their futuristic appearance is no guarantee of accuracy. Because they depend on either a microphone or a pressure transducer sewn into the cuff, it is always difficult and, in most cases impossible, to get outsize cuffs for people with large circumference arms, resulting in serious measurement errors. Unlike traditional mercury machines, anything going wrong may not be obvious, so systematically incorrect and misleading readings can be taken time and time again. Like other measuring instruments, sphygmomanometers of all

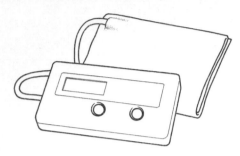

Figure 3.3 Electronic sphygmomanometer.

kinds should be compelled by law to conform to some
common minimum standard of accuracy, otherwise
different models will compete not in terms of accuracy, but
appearance and ease of use by consumers. Two published
standards are now available, one from the British
Hypertension Society and the other from the American
Association for Advancement of Medical Instrumentation
(AAAMI), but as yet nothing has been done to enforce them.
This may soon change, as a draft British Standard
specification (BS EN1060) is now being circulated for
expert appraisal. Electronic machines are constantly
improving, and once their accuracy is beyond doubt, they
will certainly replace mercury machines.

**I have seen some instruments available for BP
measurement in the pharmacy. What kind of devices are
available for self-measurement?**

The automated devices available for self-measurement all use the
same oscillometric technique. There are three categories available: devices that measure BP on the finger, the wrist and the
upper arm:

- **Finger devices**. These devices measure BP at the fingertip
  and are not recommended because of the inaccuracies
  caused by measurement distortion when the smaller blood

vessels in your hand constrict from factors such as temperature and position of your hand.

- **Wrist devices**. These devices are more accurate than fingertip measuring devices but many specialists have reservations about the correct use of these devices, particularly with regard to correct placement of the cuff on the wrist at heart level.

- **Upper arm devices**. Some of these devices can be recommended (see British Hypertension Society's website, Appendix 2). However, the recommendations that apply to BP measurement in general by means of mercury sphygmomanometry also apply to these automated devices. Appropriate cuff sizes should be used. When you take your BP, you should make sure that you have been resting for at least 5 minutes and that two separate readings are taken at least 30 seconds apart.

Accuracy of readings

What are the factors that may influence an accurate reading of BP?

There has been a great deal of research into the factors that influence and control accurate BP measurement. They can be divided into health professional-related factors, patient-related factors and instrument-related factors. Common mistakes made by health professionals when measuring BP include the use of an inappropriately short and/or narrow BP cuff. This increases both systolic and diastolic readings. It is recommended that at least 80% of the arm should be encircled by the bladder of the cuff. Sufficient time should be allowed between BP measurements. It is recommended that a minimum of two readings at any one consultation should be taken. It is also important that these two readings should be taken at least 30 seconds apart. Often the doctor or nurse may deflate the cuff too fast and inaccurately read the mercury off the sphygmomanometer. The following guides for accurate BP measurement should be followed:

- You should be seated in a quiet environment with your arm resting on a support that places the mid-point of your upper arm at the level of your heart.

- A large cuff, with the bladder encircling at least 80% of the arm, should be used.

- The lower edge of the cuff should be at least 2 cm above your elbow joint.

- The cuff should be inflated at 10 mmHg increments and the doctor or nurse should be feeling the pulse in your wrist or arm whilst doing this. A note should be made of the level at which the pulse disappears during inflation and subsequently disappears during deflation.

- The flat part ('diaphragm') of the stethoscope should be placed over the elbow joint in your arm. The bladder should be deflated steadily to 20 mm above the level found by disappearance of the pulse. Then the bladder should be deflated by 2 mm per second.

- The doctor or nurse should be listening in with the stethoscope and making note of the first appearance of repetitive sounds (these are known as 'Korotkoff sounds'). They should then take note of the mercury level at which the repetitive sounds disappear (this corresponds to your diastolic BP).

- Recording of BP should be rounded upwards to the nearest 2 mm of mercury.

The last time I visited the clinic, I had to rush in from work. Would this have altered my reading?

Yes. Many everyday activities can increase your BP. For instance, brisk walking can increase your systolic BP by up to 12 mmHg and your diastolic BP by 6 mmHg. For this reason, when you have your BP checked, it is recommended that you are resting for at least 5 minutes prior to the reading being taken. If you ran for the bus or hurried to the clinic, you should sit quietly for about half an hour before any measurement is taken. It would be worth telling the receptionist this and ask if you could delay your visit until you feel more rested.

Is the accuracy of BP measurements affected by whether I'm overweight or thin?

Measurements on people with very thin arms underestimate BP by 5–10 mmHg, however carefully they are performed. There is no way round this, and it is probably the reason why research studies generally show that high BP in very thin people appears to carry greater risks than the same levels of BP in fat people (because extremely thin people often have some other illness).

The cuff used to block flow through the artery during measurements contains an inflatable rubber bladder. This should reach round 80% of the arm circumference. In larger people, if it is too short, BP measurements may be overestimated by up to about 20 mmHg, a serious margin of error.

This is a common cause of incorrect diagnosis and unnecessary treatment. It can be avoided only by using a larger cuff. Well-equipped surgeries and hospitals have such cuffs, but doctors and nurses don't always remember to use them. Many family doctors and hospitals don't even possess outsize cuffs. If you have a larger width arm (more than about 30 cm circumference), I'm afraid you must learn (gently and courteously but firmly) to insist on the use of an outsize cuff. If you don't do this, you may easily be overtreated.

I know this is silly, but I hate going to the doctor's. Does my state of mind affect my BP measurements?

Yes it does. If you know you are anxious or frightened when you see your doctor or nurse, it is important to tell them this. Your BP measurement could be affected by what is known as 'white coat hypertension' (see questions below). You can then either arrange to have more measurements at the clinic, so that you get used to the procedure and become less anxious, or you can arrange to measure your own BP at home.

Are there any other important causes of misleading BP readings?

Apart from recent exertion, pain, fear, anger, embarrassment and so on, other important causes are:

- alcohol
- smoking
- coffee
- some kinds of medication
- a full bladder
- stress.

Large quantities of alcohol, taken slowly and steadily over months, or quickly in a binge, can raise BP substantially in many people. This is a common cause of sustained high BP in young men.

Several commonly used drugs, both prescribed and across-the-counter, tend to raise BP; these are discussed in Chapter 2. Never forget to remind your doctor or nurse what drugs you are taking, whether bought or prescribed.

If your bladder is full, your BP could rise; in people with a BP normally around 130/70 mmHg, BP may rise substantially. This can happen easily in a doctor's waiting room – if you want to go to the toilet but are afraid of losing your place in the queue, for example. It can also happen to men with benign enlargement of the prostate admitted to hospital with acute retention of urine.

Will it matter whether my BP is measured in the morning or the evening?

Most people have higher BP for a couple of hours before and after waking. In theory, BP measured in your family doctor's office early in the morning should therefore be a bit higher than if measured in the evening. In practice this seems not to happen probably because few people see their doctor within 2 hours of rising. Comparison of millions of BP measurements in a large survey in the USA showed no significant difference between measurements made in the morning and in the afternoon.

You have mentioned 'white coat hypertension'? Could you explain what this is?

This is when BP is elevated when measured during a surgery or outpatient clinic but is otherwise normal. This phenomenon usually occurs in response to the measurement of BP by a doctor or nurse. In people with normal BP, there is generally little or no difference between their BP reading at a clinic or in a surgery compared to their usual BP reading. However, in some people, substantial differences between clinic and usual BP are consistently found, with the higher readings occurring in situations where a doctor or nurse has made the BP reading. This phenomenon of white coat hypertension is more commonly seen in women and older people.

As many as 20% of people diagnosed with high BP at clinics or in surgery may have entirely normal BPs when measured during the rest of the day. In these individuals, other BP measuring techniques are recommended so that their usual pressure is accurately recorded.

So how will someone know whether my BP reading is a 'white coat hypertension' reading?

One of the reasons why BP should be taken at least twice at each consultation is to make sure that someone's BP has been given the opportunity to return to the usual or normal level if it was raised at the first reading. The white coat effect is often most pronounced when someone first enters the examination area, and declines rapidly over time. Your doctor will suspect white coat hypertension if there is a substantial difference between initial BP reading when the person enters the surgery or clinic and a subsequent reading towards the end of the consultation. Another strategy for reducing the white coat effect is to have a less 'threatening' health professional take the BP recording. Often clinics use nurses or technicians trained in BP measuring to take people's BP. The white coat effect occurs less when health professionals other than GPs take BP readings.

Ambulatory monitoring

A friend of mine had a 24-hour BP recording done. What is this and why is it performed?

What you are describing is 'ambulatory' BP monitoring. Ambulatory BP monitoring is a more rigorous and intensive way of measuring somebody's BP in whom one of the following factors may be suspected:

- when the measurement shows unusual variability in the clinic;

- where someone has 'uncontrolled hypertension' – this is high BP that has not been reduced to a target BP level after intensive drug treatment has been given;

- when people are suffering from very low BP. Low BP may affect your 'activities of daily living'. 'Postural hypotension' is a condition that can occur in such situations. This is when BP fails to adjust when a person stands up. In normal circumstances our BP increases when we stand up, but in people with postural hypotension, their BP does not increase on standing with the effect that they may feel dizzy or light-headed. In more severe cases it can cause fainting or a fall.

The most common reason for using ambulatory BP monitoring is to diagnose white coat hypertension (see questions above).

Ambulatory BP readings help distinguish between people with white coat hypertension and people who have sustained hypertension.

Ambulatory BP monitors became widely available for the first time in the late 1980s. They still depend on periodic inflation of a cuff compressing the upper arm, and thus disturb sleep seriously in some people, and may be distracting while driving a car. They don't interfere much with ordinary activities while you are sitting, but heavy work is impossible. They are usually set to measure BP at 2-hourly intervals (the best for statistical analysis). Though they are designed to be used over 48 hours, few people can tolerate them for more than 24 hours continuously.

They are a great help in sorting out 'white coat hypertension' from 'real' high BP, and thus help to avoid starting people on a lifetime of unnecessary treatment. The evidence that they provide is not always easy to interpret because all the important evidence that we have on the value and limitations of long-term treatment for high BP at various levels is based on surgery readings by means of mercury sphygmomanometers.

What are the advantages and disadvantages of ambulatory BP monitoring?

Ambulatory BP monitoring permits the non-invasive measurement of BP over a prolonged period of time (usually 24 hours). It was first developed as a research tool in the 1960s and 1970s – it has now become a popular way of assessing the average BP reading. Its advantages are that it provides a more representative estimate of someone's BP reading compared to isolated clinical readings. In addition, BP values derived from ambulatory readings are better markers for the risk of possible organ damage in the future caused by hypertension (what is called 'prognostic information') than usual BP readings at the surgery or clinic.

The main disadvantage is that ambulatory BP monitoring is an expensive technology. It also requires specialist involvement, as interpretation of ambulatory readings can be complex and requires specialist training.

Monitoring at home

A friend of mine has an electronic BP monitor at home. What are the advantages and disadvantages of self-measuring BP?

Automated electronic devices provide timed printouts of BP and remove many of the sources of error associated with conventional BP measurement. The critical point is to make sure that any electronic device that you use when measuring your own BP has been validated against a conventional mercury sphygmo-manometer. You can check the British Hypertension Society website for details of validated machines (see Appendix 2).

There are various points to remember when taking your own BP reading:

- Sit quietly and comfortably without distractions in a warm room throughout the procedure.

- Your measurement arm (normally the left arm in right-handed people) should be supported (usually by a table) at about the same level as your heart (the level of the nipple in men). You'll need a small cushion or a book under your arm to ensure this. If your arm is far above or below your heart, you'll get a false reading.

- Make sure you have no tight clothing above the cuff. If you just roll up your sleeve, it may be so tight that it puts pressure on the brachial artery itself, and thus gives a false low BP measurement. At least while you're learning how to use the device, it's wise to remove all clothing from the arm before you begin the measurement.

Electronic monitoring devices come with an instruction book, which nowadays is usually adequate. As they vary in how fully they are automated, and in the various symbols and icons that they use on their displays, you will need to read this instruction book to fully understand what you are doing. Most of them have some sort of automatic inflation of the cuff, followed by automatic deflation, triggered by recognition of systolic pressure. The rate of deflation may or may not be variable. If it is, set it to the slowest rate possible and don't speed this up later, even if it makes the procedure more comfortable. If it is not variable, check the time it takes to go from, say, 140 mmHg to 80 mmHg against the seconds hand on your watch. This should take 1 minute and 20 seconds. If it takes less than a minute, don't buy or use the machine.

Electronic monitoring devices recognize systolic and diastolic pressures either through a microphone, which recognizes the appearance and disappearance of regular tapping sounds, or through a transducer, which recognizes a pulse wave. Transducers are more efficient (but more expensive), and less prone to pick up extraneous signals. In both cases, the part of the cuff containing the sensor must be placed accurately over the brachial pulse. Failure to do this is the commonest cause of inaccurate or failed BP reading. The brachial pulse can be felt along the crease of your inner arm. It lies on the inside part of your biceps tendon (Figure 3.4).

Virtually all electronic monitoring devices measure your pulse as well as BP. These are useful indicators of your state of mind while you are measuring your BP. Rates over about 80 beats a minute suggest some anxiety.

The common causes of false measurements at home are anxiety, fear, anger, pain, embarrassment and cold. If you feel relaxed and are not distracted by other things going on, you can be reasonably confident that the pressures you record are

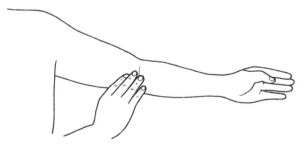

Figure 3.4 Locating the brachial artery pulse.

correct. If you really cannot relax, and always feel anxious when measuring your own BP, say so, because this factor needs to be taken into account by your doctor. Cold is a powerful raiser of BP, and if you have come in from a frosty winter's day, take half an hour or so to warm up before measuring your BP.

Are there any situations where electronic devices are not recommended?

In some situations the oscillometric technique that electronic monitors use is not reliable and accurate in people with specific problems. The commonest cause is in people who have an irregular pulse, most notably atrial fibrillation. This is a condition where the upper chambers of the heart, the atria, 'fibrillate' rather than beat regularly. Atrial fibrillation is not life-threatening as the main chambers of the heart, the ventricles, continue to beat regularly. Atrial fibrillation is associated with a greater risk of suffering a stroke and you will probably be given a blood-thinning drug either in the form of aspirin or warfarin (see Chapter 6). Atrial fibrillation can be detected by the doctor taking an electrocardiogram (ECG) reading.

A friend of mine has been told that BP readings need to be adjusted when electronic devices as opposed to mercury sphygmomanometers are used. What does this mean?

It is recognized that repeated daytime measurements of BP produces systematically lower BP readings compared with isolated surgery or clinic readings. Because of this phenomenon, treatment thresholds (the BP level for initiating treatment) and target threshold (the target BP which should be aimed at when taking BP-lowering drugs) need to be adjusted downwards when the doctor makes a decision based on self-measuring electronic devices or ambulatory BP readings. The general recommended difference between clinic and daytime mean BP readings is thought to be about 12/7 mmHg.

What are the advantages and disadvantages of taking my own BP readings by means of an electronic device?

The advantages of taking your own readings are that multiple readings can be obtained over a prolonged period of time allowing better definition of your true BP. As no medical personnel are involved, distortion due to the white coat effect is far less likely. The disadvantages are that many of these devices are inaccurate and may produce false readings. This leads to incorrect interpretation of the BP measurements from the device (the British Hypertension Society's website lists electronic machines that have been checked and validated – see Appendix 2). Another reason to take your BP concerns monitoring of your BP once you have started BP treatment. Some people find this form of self-monitoring reassuring. However, there are two caveats that should be remembered: firstly, self-readings need to be adjusted downwards by 12/7 mmHg so as to be consistent with surgery/clinic readings; secondly, there is very little evidence that home self-measurement of BP is an effective way to help people reach target BP and may cause unnecessary anxiety when spuriously 'high' or 'low' readings are read.

4
Non-pharmacological treatment

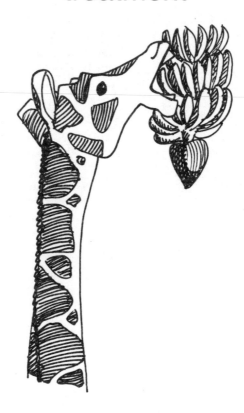

Changing your lifestyle, including diet, exercise and smoking, will help to lessen the risk of heart attacks and strokes. This chapter looks at ways of changing your lifestyle when you find that your BP is raised.

Can I bring my BP down to normal without taking drugs?

The answer depends on how high your average BP is. Generally speaking, if after several measurements over a period of 4–6 weeks, your BP remains raised (averages more than 150/90 mmHg) and your risk of heart attack or stroke is high when estimated from a cardiovascular risk chart, you will need to consider options to reduce both your BP and overall cardiovascular risk. As mentioned in earlier chapters, BP alone is only one of several risk factors that determine your likelihood of suffering a heart attack or stroke. It makes sense to address your overall cardiovascular risk by changing all your risk factors.

Cholesterol levels

The following questions explain all about cholesterol but there is more about its treatment alongside treatment for BP in Chapter 6.

I am going to have a cholesterol test soon. What is cholesterol and why is it important?

Cholesterol is an essential component of all body cells and of many important circulating chemicals in the blood (hormones). It is formed from many different sorts of fats and oils in what you eat, including cholesterol itself, which is present in large quantities in some foods such as egg yolks, liver, kidneys, meats and fish roes. It is then distributed where it is needed in the body. If there is a surplus, most of this is stored in the liver, but some remains circulating in the blood.

Blood cholesterol concentration is now measured in millimoles per litre (normally written as mmol/litre), except in North America, which still uses milligrams per decilitre (normally written as mg/dl). This value varies between countries (mainly because of differences in fat intake), from an average below 4 mmol in China, to nearly 6 mmol in the UK. For individuals, otherwise normal people may have blood cholesterols varying from about 3.5 mmol to about 15 mmol.

The reason the concentration of blood cholesterol matters is that the higher it is, the more it is deposited as waxy plaques on the walls of coronary arteries supplying blood to the heart, to brain arteries, and to the aorta and leg arteries, which then causes narrowing of the walls. The narrowing tends to cause clotting and thus partial or complete destruction of the organs supplied by these arteries.

Scientific studies in many countries over many years have confirmed a close connection between average levels of blood cholesterol and coronary heart disease in people aged under 65 in whole populations, and a somewhat less close connection for individuals. There is no doubt whatever that, in all societies where average blood cholesterol is low, coronary heart disease is rare, or that, in all societies where it is high, coronary heart disease is common. This remains true even if other risk factors for coronary heart disease are common in low-cholesterol societies, or low in high-cholesterol societies. For example, although high BP and heavy smoking are extremely common in China, resulting in many strokes, coronary heart disease remains rare; whereas in western countries where both smoking and uncontrolled high BP have become much less common, but average blood cholesterol has not fallen, as in Sweden, coronary heart disease remains common.

The media talks about good and bad kinds of blood cholesterol? What are these?

When doctors talk loosely about 'blood cholesterol' they normally mean total cholesterol, but this is actually made up of three parts. If you leave about 10 ml of blood standing in a glass tube until it has clotted, the cholesterol it contains becomes easily visible as a cloudy yellowish substance, occupying the top quarter or so of the tube. It looks like what it is, a sort of fat. If you put this in a high speed centrifuge, the yellow stuff separates out according to molecular size and weight, into three parts:

- high density lipoprotein (HDL)
- low density lipoprotein (LDL), and
- very low density lipoprotein (VLDL) cholesterol.

LDL and VLDL cholesterol are 'bad' cholesterol, the source of waxy plaques on the walls of the aorta, coronary arteries, brain arteries and leg arteries that ultimately weaken or block these vessels, and cause organ damage by clotting or bleeding. HDL cholesterol, on the other hand, is 'good'. Many studies have shown that concentrations of HDL cholesterol above about 1.5 mmol make coronary heart disease less likely, and low levels (below 1 mmol) make it more likely. This is probably because HDL is the form in which cholesterol is transported in blood before storage in the liver or excretion in bile. LDL and VLDL are thus measures of a tendency to harmful deposition of cholesterol in artery walls, whereas HDL is a measure of beneficial storage of cholesterol in liver or excretion in bile.

As LDL and VLDL together usually account for about 80% of total blood cholesterol, total blood cholesterol can generally be accepted as a valid though approximate measure of 'bad' cholesterol, while ignoring the contribution from 'good' cholesterol. Most laboratories now report both HDL and total cholesterol and some of the risk charts estimate cardiovascular risk based on the HDL/total cholesterol ratio (discussed under *Diagnosis* in Chapter 2).

Sophisticated measurements of blood fats (lipids) often also include triglyceride, the form in which fat is first absorbed from the gut. Except in the special case of what is known as 'inherited familial hypercholesterolaemia' (see question below), measurement of triglyceride is rarely of practical value. High values are commonly associated with fatness, or high alcohol consumption, or both. Once these are taken into account, high triglyceride is not a good predictor of whether you will have a heart attack.

Measurements of cholesterol fractions and triglyceride are obviously more complex and costly for the laboratory, but it is also more bother for you because, while total cholesterol and HDL cholesterol can be measured accurately on any sample of blood, LDL, VLDL and triglyceride can be measured accurately only after a minimum fasting period of 12 hours, during which no food or drinks other than water can be taken.

What are the benefits of treating my high cholesterol level as well as my high BP?

Raised cholesterol ('dyslipidaemia') is another risk factor for coronary heart disease. There is a two-fold increase in the risk of suffering a heart attack or stroke in people who have raised total and LDL cholesterol and low levels of HDL, compared to people without such findings. The relationship between high triglyceride levels and future risk of cardiovascular disease (particularly heart attack) is less clear cut. Reducing your cholesterol levels with drugs will be discussed in more detail in Chapter 6, but the key is that your overall risk of heart attack or stroke is calculated, as drug treatment can be beneficial, but greater benefit is gained from treatment of people with high risk.

My father has high blood cholesterol. Is it likely that I will have high levels as well?

Yes, unfortunately very much so. Regardless of inheritance, people on an extremely low-fat diet, for example the poorest people in China, cannot have high blood cholesterol levels, but once people are rich enough to eat as much as they want of the cheaper foods available, the main determinant of individual blood cholesterol levels is not personal diet, but personal chemistry, and this is strongly inherited. Some people can eat a lot of fats and oils without getting either a high blood cholesterol or cholesterol plaques in their arteries; others are not so lucky, and the main difference lies in their genes.

A few people (about 1 per 500) have inherited genes for very high blood cholesterol from one parent ('heterozygous hyper-cholesterolaemia'), and even fewer (less than 1 per 1000) have inherited them from both parents ('homozygous hyper-cholesterolaemia'). Homozygotes mostly die from coronary heart attacks before they reach 30. Heterozygotes have a peak risk of coronary heart attacks between the ages of 20 and 39 but, if they survive this, subsequently have about the same risk as the general population. All these people have blood total cholesterol levels around 9–15 mmol, with very high LDL and VLDL cholesterol levels, very low HDL cholesterol levels, and usually very high triglyceride levels. They all deserve specialist investigation and initial counselling and treatment at a special lipid clinic. As well as skilled dietary advice, they invariably need cholesterol-lowering medication. 'Familial hypercholesterolaemia' should be sought for in the surviving relatives (including children and grandchildren) whenever anyone has a fatal or non-fatal coronary heart attack under the age of 50.

The vast majority of people with 'high blood cholesterol' are not in this category; they simply eat what most of us eat, and suffer the consequences of any diet in which 40% or more of all energy is consumed as fat.

Can I do anything to increase 'good' HDL blood cholesterol?

Yes. HDL cholesterol is increased by exercise, by stopping smoking, and by drinking alcohol. The latter is possibly the main reason for low death rates from premature coronary heart disease in France, but correspondingly high death rates for cirrhosis of the liver more than make up for this!

Diet

Cholesterol-lowering by diet

Can high blood cholesterol really be reduced by changing what we eat?

There is good evidence that the big differences in average blood cholesterol levels (and consequent differences in premature coronary death rates) between different countries depend on differences in what people eat, and that when nations as a whole eat less fat or take more exercise (for example, the USA and Finland), average blood cholesterol levels fall, and so do coronary death rates. Unfortunately, efforts put into the same changes in personal diets have been less effective.

So what should I be doing with my diet if my cholesterol is raised?

There have been several clinical studies that have evaluated low-fat diets on cholesterol reduction and risk of heart attack and stroke. Modest reductions of approximately 5% in total cholesterol over several months were achieved in these studies. There is an association between the intensity of lowering your cholesterol intake by means of a diet and subsequent reduction in cholesterol levels. More intense, low-fat diets result in greater reduction in cholesterol than less intense diets. These intense cholesterol-lowering diets have contributed to a small reduction in total mortality. Many of these studies lasted only around 6 months, but those that lasted at least 2 years provided stronger evidence for protection from cardiovascular disease, reducing the risk by about 25%.

Our general advice would be to try to reduce your dietary fat intake in conjunction with other non-drug therapies, but to be realistic in recognizing that dietary modification of your fat intake is difficult to achieve.

Is garlic good for high BP or high blood cholesterol?

Garlic has no significant effect on high BP, and there is conflicting evidence that it reduces blood cholesterol. Some studies have shown that large quantities of fresh (not powdered) garlic used in cooking reduce LDL cholesterol ('bad' cholesterol) by an average of 12% (about 0.7 mmol) but have no effect on HDL cholesterol ('good' cholesterol); other studies have shown no effect on cholesterol lowering.

Other dietary help

Will eating a low-fat, high fruit and vegetable diet help to reduce my BP?

Healthy eating is a broad term for a change of diet to increased intake in fresh fruit and vegetables as well as an increase in low-fat foods. In terms of reducing BP there is good evidence that a low-fat, high fruit and vegetable diet does reduce BP in people with no history of cardiovascular disease. Reductions in BP have been in the region of 3 mmHg diastolic and 5 mmHg systolic BP. Although these are not as large reductions as for other non-drug activities such as exercise, if you keep to this diet they will be worthwhile and reduce your chance of suffering a stroke or heart attack. There is some good advice on eating more and varied fruit and vegetables on the Blood Pressure Association's website (see Appendix 2).

Should I eat more fibre?

'Dietary fibre' usually means everything in your food that you cannot digest, and therefore is excreted. It includes lots of important materials that are not fibrous at all, such as gums, which affect both the way in which food is absorbed, and the quantity you want to eat before you begin to feel full and tired of chewing.

As well as breakfast cereals and wholemeal bread, all fruit and vegetables have a high fibre content, although how much you actually get depends on whether you cook them or eat them raw. Routine addition of sodium bicarbonate to keep vegetables green rapidly destroys their fibre content, as does prolonged boiling. Steaming and microwaving vegetables are the best cooking methods. Fresh fruit and raw salads are ideal.

Pulses (peas, beans, lentils, etc.) have the highest fibre content of any cooked vegetables. Increasing the fibre content of your diet by eating more wholemeal bread, fruit and vegetables is one of the most effective steps you can take in any reduced-fat, weight-reducing, and cholesterol-lowering diet.

The nurse in our practice said that I should try and eat a 'healthy diet'. What is meant by a healthy diet? Should it include foods that are eaten in the Mediterranean region?

Most of the good results in studies have been due to changes in diet involving eating a minimum of five portions of fruit and vegetables per day. Often these studies have been delivered through health promotion advice from nurses so that people's new eating habits are monitored and reinforced.

There have been no studies specifically addressing the issue of BP lowering by increasing fish intake or changing your diet to a Mediterranean-type diet. However, the benefits of high fish diets have been demonstrated in other situations, particularly in the lowering of risk for heart attack (myocardial infarction). The benefit of changing to a Mediterranean diet, which consists of bread, fruit, vegetables and fish, with less meat and replacement of butter and cream with olive or rapeseed oils, has not been shown to be associated with reductions in BP levels but there is good evidence that diet does reduce your risk of heart attack or stroke.

So, are there any particular types of fish that could help to reduce BP?

Fatty fish, such as mackerel, herrings, salmon and trout, have an important protective effect against coronary heart disease, and are an important part of any prudent diet for people with high BP. The effect is probably through what are known as omega-3 fish oils, which can be taken as capsules. They reduce blood levels of triglyceride, the form in which fat is transported from the gut to the liver.

I have heard that eggs and dairy foods are bad for you, but I am a non-meat eater and like eggs and milk. Are these OK?

Strict vegetarian diets can easily become deficient in protein, which is essential for building new cells. Fish, eggs and cheese are important possible sources of protein as well as variety for most vegetarians. They are not eaten by strict vegetarians (vegans), who must rely on pulses (beans and peas) and nuts as their most protein-rich foods.

Egg yolks are high in cholesterol, but as a source of high blood cholesterol they are no more important than other foods containing animal fats, which, when digested, are changed into body cholesterol. A good diet should contain not more than two eggs a week, but if you cut down on other fats, you can eat more.

All cheeses except cottage cheese contain large amounts of salt, so cheeses have to be virtually eliminated from any serious low-salt diet. They also contain a lot of saturated fat, which raises blood cholesterol. The same applies to butter, except that you can easily get low-salt butter. For reasons that so far remain unexplained, people who drink a lot of milk tend to have lower blood cholesterol levels than people who drink little or none. Evidence for this is consistent and apparently reliable. However, milk does contain a lot of salt, and has to be restricted in low-salt diets.

What about increasing my potassium intake? I've been told that bananas and other fruits are the most effective way of doing this. Will they decrease my BP?

You are correct. The best way to increase potassium is to eat more fresh fruit and vegetables. However, a potassium balance is maintained within a fairly narrow range by physiological mechanisms in the kidney. There is some evidence that increasing your potassium intake by about 200 mg, roughly equivalent to the amount contained in five bananas, does reduce BP by small amounts.

Our advice to people is that increases in potassium intake are consistent with increasing a fruit and vegetable intake. Somewhat like the salt issue, we think that there is unlikely to be any harm in increasing your fruit and vegetable intake, but you should be realistic about the size of benefit in terms of lowering your BP. Increasing the potassium intake in the form of bananas or other fruits to a substantial extent should be cautioned in people with a history of kidney problems. In these people, excretion of excessive potassium can sometimes become impaired.

What about taking multivitamins and antioxidants, do they help?

Until recently there was a great deal of excitement about the potential for taking vitamin supplements and antioxidants in reducing risk for heart attacks and strokes both in people with and without high BP. Unfortunately, randomized trials of vitamin supplementation and antioxidants have been disappointing and have failed to show substantial benefit.

We routinely tell people who ask whether vitamin supplementation is worthwhile that there is no evidence to suggest that it will reduce either their BP or their risk of having a stroke or heart attack.

My wife is a vegetarian. Would a vegetarian diet help me to lower my BP?

Yes it would. BP is on average lower in vegetarians than in meat-eaters, and BP falls in people on a vegetarian diet who have BP high enough to need treatment, though rarely enough to avoid any need for BP-lowering drugs. We have good evidence that potassium (which comes mainly from fruit and vegetables – see question above) reduces BP, and this may be the main way in which a vegetarian diet works.

Salt intake

I have always put salt on my food. I am now told that I have to cut this out. Will this be an effective way of lowering my BP?

The relationship between salt intake and BP levels is a contentious and controversial subject. Population studies comparing the effects of consumption of salt and BP in different countries or regions have shown clearly that, in countries where there is greater average salt intake, there is a higher risk of stroke and other cardiovascular disease.

High BP does not exist at all, nor does average BP rise with age, in some tribes in Brazil and Papua–New Guinea where salt intake is at the bare minimum essential for life (less than 15 mmol sodium a day), about one-tenth of the present average intake in the UK (about 150 mmol a day). On the other hand, in countries with very high sodium intakes, such as rural Portugal where average sodium intake is about twice that in the UK (300 mmol a day), or rural northern Japan where the intake is more than two and a half times the UK intake (400 mmol a day), both high BP and stroke are extremely common.

Studies show that, compared to usual diet, low-salt diets modestly reduce BP levels in the region of 1–2 mmHg systolic and 0.5 mmHg diastolic BP. In these studies of salt reduction, very few people have been followed up to see whether they suffer later from a heart problem; thus all the information relates to BP control rather than probability of suffering a stroke or heart attack. Another issue is that the changes in salt intake in some of these studies were very intensive, requiring substantial alteration in the usual diet. Whether such changes in diet can be sustained outside of clinical trial settings is the subject of different opinions in the high BP research community. The main recommendation is that reducing salt intake is worthwhile, particularly in the elderly or those people already taking BP-lowering drugs. Reduction of salt intake in conjunction with changes in diet and increasing exercise may allow some people to achieve a sufficient reduction in their BP to allow them to stop taking BP-lowering drugs. However, this assumes that reductions in salt are not accompanied by a rise in fat intake. This may happen easily if low-salt food seems tasteless.

How should I go about modifying the salt intake in my diet?

The main source of sodium in most foods is sodium chloride, ordinary salt. This is present not only in added cooking salt or table salt, but also in such usually unsuspected high-sodium foods as milk, cheese and bread, and in virtually all tinned or ready pre-pared foods such as most breakfast cereals, sausages, burgers, pizzas and soups. A diet sufficiently low in sodium to reduce BP, with sodium intake reduced to about half normal at 60–70 mmol a day, must virtually eliminate all these foods, as well as more obvious ones like kippers, bacon, olives, hummus and Marmite.

There are two secrets of successful reduction of dietary sodium:

- The first is to reduce salt intake slowly, taking 3 months or more to reach your target. After a few months you find that your sense of taste has more or less permanently changed, and normally salted foods become quite unpleasant. Although there will still be many delicious foods that you cannot eat, what you can eat will (eventually) start to taste good again.

- The second secret is to include the whole family in the diet, so that the whole meal can be cooked in the same way. As high BP runs so strongly in families, this is a good idea anyway.

If you follow a moderately low-sodium diet of this kind, and if you have mildly raised BP in the diastolic range 90–95 mmHg, you may not need any medication. If it is much higher than this, you may need lower doses, or fewer different drugs, than you would on your usual diet. A dietitian will be able to help you adjust your salt intake. There is some good advice on how to cut your salt on the Blood Pressure Association's website (see Appendix 2).

Alcohol

I have heard that drinking alcohol is now considered good for you! I always thought that too much can be bad. Which is right?

There is a relationship between high alcohol consumption and higher BP levels. High alcohol consumption is clearly associated with a substantial risk of having high BP that requires treatment.

Regular heavy drinking raises BP, particularly in young men. This response varies, and is substantial in some people, so much so that, in many young men with diastolic pressures consistently over 100 mmHg, BP may fall to normal without medication, once drinking is reduced to a pint or two of beer each day. High alcohol intake is a common cause of treatment failure and, if your BP refuses to fall despite apparently adequate treatment, you should think about what you are drinking. Heavy drinking in one session (bingeing) can cause a rapid though brief rise in BP, which may precipitate a stroke in older people.

Very heavy drinking (15 pints a day or more for a man) increases coronary risk. However, there is consistent evidence that moderate drinking (up to 2 pints of beer or 4 glasses of wine a day for men, half that for women) reduces risk of heart attack, probably through effects on blood cholesterol and clotting factors.

I know I drink more than the recommended number of units per day of alcohol. Should I reduce my alcohol consumption? Will this be effective in bringing down my BP?

Our advice to people who drink over the recommended levels of 21 and 28 units per week for women and men, respectively, is to reduce their alcohol consumption. There is a reduction in coronary heart disease associated with modest alcohol consumption (less than 2 units of alcohol a day), so drinking a glass of wine each day really is good for you! However, in people who have high BP sufficient to warrant the doctor to consider prescribing drug treatment, reducing alcohol consumption is an effective way of reducing high BP and avoiding having to take BP-lowering drugs. Consumption of one or two drinks of alcohol per day is probably safe and may be protective, but any more than this is associated with an increase in BP and consequent risk of heart attack or stroke. There is some good advice on alcohol and BP on the Blood Pressure Association's website (see Appendix 2).

Smoking

I am a heavy smoker and have been told to stop. What are the benefits of stopping smoking?

Smoking is strongly associated with increased overall heart attack and stroke risk, cancers and respiratory disease, and has a strong relationship with overall mortality rates. For example, middle-aged smokers are three times more likely to die early than their non-smoking counterparts. There is also a strong dose-response relationship: the more cigarettes you smoke, the greater your risk of cancer, cardiovascular problems and death.

For these reasons, quitting smoking is a good idea. There are several smoking-quitting strategies that are known to be effective. Several studies have shown that counselling and nicotine replacement (in the form of a patch, gum or nasal spray) are effective in helping people to quit smoking.

In people who stop smoking, risk of cardiovascular problems, cancer and death falls substantially. It appears that for people who are ex-smokers, their risk falls gradually to a risk level between lifelong smokers and people who have never smoked in the past.

There is also a newer and effective drug available to people in whom nicotine replacement has not worked – buproprion (Zyban), a form of antidepressant.

Our advice is that quitting smoking is probably the most important thing you can do to reduce your overall risk of heart attack or stroke whether you have hypertension or not. Community counselling services offered in conjunction with nicotine replacement or buproprion treatment are available on the NHS. You should ask your doctor to arrange referral to these support services. Alternatively, write to Action on Smoking and Health (ASH), at their address given in Appendix 2.

So will stopping smoking reduce my BP as well as my risk of heart attack or stroke?

No, but for most people with high BP who smoke, stopping smoking reduces the risk of coronary heart attacks more than does reducing BP itself, particularly in younger people; it also greatly reduces the risk of obstructed leg arteries, cancer of the lung, throat, larynx, pancreas and bladder, stops further deterioration of chronic bronchitis and airways obstruction, and somewhat reduces your risk of stroke. All this alone makes stopping smoking very worthwhile.

If I can't stop smoking, will that make treatment for high BP ineffective?

Generally, no. Benefit from treatment is greatest in people at highest risk. As people who continue smoking are at much higher risk than those who stop, or never started, they actually benefit more from treatment. The greatest probable health gains are from both stopping smoking and reducing BP.

Which is most important, stopping smoking or controlling high BP?

Smoking is a bigger and more completely reversible risk factor than high BP, except in a small minority of people with very severe high BP, usually with diastolic pressures well over 120 mmHg.

Smoking is not a cause of high BP, but it greatly increases its consequent risks. If you have high BP already, your risk of a heart attack is increased three times by smoking up to about 50 years of age, and doubled after that age. Heart attacks in people under 45 happen almost entirely in smokers.

Smoking is a very powerful risk factor in its own right, not only for coronary heart disease and stroke, but also for cancer as mentioned above, and for asthma and other obstructive lung diseases. Unlike all other risk factors, it also affects your family and friends, because they are subjected to passive smoking, and the example you set to your children is poor.

I quite like smoking cigars or a pipe. Are these safer substitutes for cigarettes?

Generally no. People who have smoked cigars or a pipe all their lives, and have never smoked cigarettes, rarely inhale tobacco smoke and are therefore at lower risk of all the consequences of smoking, other than cancer of the mouth and throat, but very few such people exist. Virtually all cigarette smokers inhale, whether consciously or unconsciously. If they change to pipe or cigar smoking, they continue to inhale (often unconsciously and with furious denials, refuted by tests for carbon monoxide levels). Their loads of both nicotine and carbon monoxide (the main reasons why smoking promotes heart disease) and of tobacco tar (the main reason why smoking promotes lung cancer) are even greater in cigar and most pipe smokers, than in cigarette smokers.

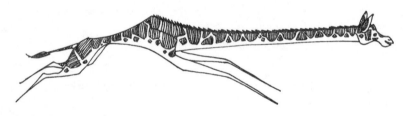

Exercise

If I start an exercise programme now, what will that achieve?

Although the immediate effect of exercise is to raise BP, the long-term effect of regular exercise is to reduce BP by about 5/3 mmHg (i.e. 5 mmHg systolic and 3 mmHg diastolic BB).

Regular exercise also reduces a wide range of important risk factors for coronary heart disease and stroke: it reduces harmful LDL and VLDL blood cholesterol (see the section above on cholesterol), raises protective HDL blood cholesterol, and reduces the blood clotting factor fibrinogen. It reduces bodyweight by increasing energy output, and helps you to keep to a healthy diet by raising morale. In the same way, regular exercise often helps people to stop smoking.

Exercising more helps to reduce your coronary heart and stroke risk by between 20–40% compared with those people who live sedentary lives. Their risk of cardiovascular disease would be lowered by increasing their levels of activity. High levels of exercising are associated with about 3 extra lives saved per 1000. The benefits of exercise can be seen significantly on a long-term basis.

I do some brisk walking. How much would benefit me?

There have been many studies assessing various type of exercise including walking/jogging, cycling, swimming or combinations of exercise. The ideal time is about half an hour to an hour, three times per week. These levels of activity reduce BP levels in both people with high and normal BP. The size of benefit in exercising compared to non-exercising groups is a lowering of BP in the region of 5 mmHg systolic and 3 mmHg diastolic BP. There is some evidence that exercise is of greater benefit in people with higher initial BP readings.

How hard and often should I exercise?

A lot depends on how much you exercise now. We would not recommend that you start taking vigorous exercise when you have previously been living a sedentary life. However, even moderate exercise, equivalent to brisk walking, helps towards improved fitness, wellbeing and reduction in BP. Our advice is that, if you've been leading a previously sedentary life, you should consult your doctor to make sure that you're not overambitious to start with. You should start moderate exercise for a minimum of half an hour, three times per week. You can then build up your exercise programme depending on how you feel.

The first rule for all successful exercise programmes is for people to do what they want, what interests them. A serious problem for many people is that many forms of sustained exercise are boring. You are far more likely to establish regular new habits and stick to them, if you enjoy what you are doing.

- Cycling is an excellent exercise for everyone except people with back problems, although even they can manage if they get a really wide, well-sprung seat and high handlebars.

- Swimming is an ideal form of exercise for older people or people with arthritis, because your body is weightless and movements may become almost painless when you are immersed in water. If you don't know how to swim, ask at your local pool for beginners' classes – most have then for all ages. Learning to swim properly will keep your head in alignment with your spine – swimming with your head out of the water can create neck problems.

People with established high BP should avoid extremely vigorous or competitive sports such as squash, and static exercises like weight-lifting and push-ups, all of which may raise BP for a short time to dangerous levels. Jogging, long-distance running and non-competitive cycling are all suitable forms of exercise providing you start slowly, train up gradually, and generally use some common sense. A local gym might be able to help you work out a suitable regimen for you.

Could I harm myself from too much exercise?

Muscular skeletal strains, sprains and other injuries are the commonest problems associated with people who have previously been sedentary. We recommend that exercise should be graded, started at a low level of intensity and built up over a period of time.

There is a small risk of sudden death associated with strenuous activity but, in absolute terms, this is very rare. It happens in less than 1 per 10,000 person-hours of exercise. Sudden death is greatest among people who have been previously sedentary. Risk of suffering a heart attack is substantially greater in relative terms in people who were previously sedentary, so start slowly and gradually build up your exercise programme. There is more advice on exercise and BP on the Blood Pressure Association's website (see Appendix 2).

Weight loss

I am rather overweight and keep meaning to do something about it. Will losing weight help to reduce my BP?

There is considerable evidence that losing weight is associated with important reductions in BP in obese people. Reductions of 10% of bodyweight can be achieved by motivated people by reducing calorie intakes to 450–1500 kilocalories per day. The size of benefit is 3 mmHg systolic and 3 mmHg diastolic BP reduction.

A more important benefit is that, in people already taking BP-lowering drugs, weight reduction is associated with a lower dose and fewer BP-lowering drugs being needed to control their BP to target levels. More important still is the effect of weight reduction in reducing your risk of diabetes to which people with raised BP are especially prone. There is some good advice on weight loss on the Blood Pressure Association's website (see Appendix 2).

Would it help if I joined a weight-losing group?

We routinely recommend weight loss to overweight and obese people. Such a strategy has a clear benefit in controlling BP. However, many people find weight loss a difficult target to achieve. We advise people to join WeightWatchers or other such organizations, as there is good evidence that losing weight with a group is more effective than trying to do it by yourself.

Commercial weight-losing groups like WeightWatchers are well known, and available in almost all towns. If you join one of these, you are more likely to lose weight and maintain your loss. The standard of dietary advice is probably better than you will get from the average family doctor; however, they are expensive enough to be out of reach for many people's pockets. Equally good results have been achieved by non-commercial voluntary groups, often based on NHS health centres or group practices. Most have been started by local enthusiasts, people as well as Practice Nurses, Health Visitors or Community Dietitians. If the sort of group you think you need does not exist locally, and you fancy the task of starting one, you should get in touch with others who have real past experience of doing this. Dietitians at your local hospital, or your Community Dietitians if there are any near you, will probably be able to help you.

How exactly does weight or weight loss affect BP?

Body growth mainly depends on ultimate stature, i.e. adult body size and shape. In people who have been well nourished in childhood, this depends almost entirely on inheritance but, if childhood nutrition is poor, full potential inherited stature may not be reached. Even in a comparatively rich country like Britain, there are still big differences in average height between income groups, and these differences are actually greater now than they were in the 1930s. Growth hormone is an important determinant of BP in adolescence, and is also one of several determinants of Type 2 (non-insulin-dependent) diabetes in middle age, the others being inheritance and overweight.

Although the connections between causes of high BP and causes of diabetes are not yet fully understood, they are certainly important for a large proportion of both groups. People with high BP are more likely to get diabetes later on, people with diabetes are more likely to get high BP, and both are powerful causes of stroke and coronary heart disease. For these reasons throughout this book, although it is supposed to be about high BP, diabetes keeps cropping up. Nature has little respect for labels. There is evidence that undernutrition during fetal development or infancy, followed by overnutrition in adolescence or adult life, may be a common and important cause of high BP and diabetes.

The weight clinic that I attend is always talking about Body Mass Index or BMI. What exactly is this?

We can rank people for weight despite varying height by using the Body Mass Index (BMI) formula:

$$BMI = \frac{\text{weight in kilograms}}{\text{height in metres}^2} \quad \text{or} \quad \frac{kg}{m^2}$$

Your BMI is in the normal range if it is between 20 and 25. For example, if you weigh 80 kg and are 2 metres high, your BMI would be 20. People below BMI 20 are underweight, and above BMI 25 are overweight. Over 30 is classed as obesity. The rise in death rates for obesity rises rapidly from a BMI of 30, so this is when dietary control of weight is particularly important.

My weight is spread around my middle. Does this matter?

BMI is a useful rough guide to desirable weight for height, but it takes no account of good evidence that body shape is more important than weight-for-height alone. Overweight people whose body fat is concentrated around the middle are more likely to have high BP, and are at higher risk of coronary disease, than overweight people whose body fat is mainly in their arms, legs, breasts and buttocks. The best way to measure this is to divide belly girth by hip girth, both at their widest point: a healthy result is less than 1.00. Coronary risk rises in people whose belly girth is greater than their hip girth – the beer-drinker's belly.

My doctor has advised that addressing all non-drug treatments simultaneously – weight loss, salt reduction, more exercise and less alcohol – is the most effective way of reducing my BP. This seems like hard work. Is it worth it?

Yes it is, though you're quite correct that it will require quite a lot of effort. A recent randomized trial in the USA of obese (BMI greater than 30), middle-aged patients (average age 50) with moderately raised BP showed that sustained changes in lifestyle including increasing exercise, losing weight (loss of about 5 kg on average), moderating alcohol consumption and changing diet (reducing salt intake and increasing fruit and vegetable intake) resulted in a reduction of about 4 mmHg systolic blood pressure on average. Though non-drug treatment does not produce falls in BP as substantial as drug treatment (see Chapter 5), it does have the advantage that other risk factors are simultaneously altered, resulting in an overall reduction of cardiovascular risk. Non-drug treatment is highly beneficial whatever age you are.

5
Treatment with drugs

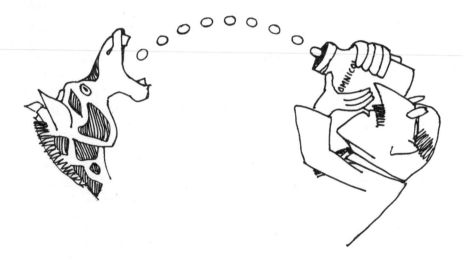

Having to take drugs for high BP is now common for many people in the UK and in other developed countries: about one-fifth of people aged 70 or more take BP-lowering drugs. This chapter will discuss the benefits of and problems associated with BP-lowering drugs.

The goal of drug treatment with BP-lowering drugs is to:

- decrease the risk of cardiovascular disease (heart attack and stroke), associated with raised BP;

- control any risk of other cardiovascular risk factors that may be present such as raised cholesterol, diabetes, left ventricular hypertrophy, and other conditions that may need other drugs, aside from blood pressure-lowering drugs;

- improve your quality of life.

The choice of drug treatment will be 'tailored' to maximize the benefits and minimize the side effects according to your profile of these other risk factors, preferences for treatment and your circumstances.

There seems to be a lot of different drugs on the market for high BP. Are the benefits and risks of these drugs well established?

Drug treatment for high BP is probably one of the best researched areas in medical practice. Thousands of people have participated in clinical trials comparing BP-lowering drugs against a 'dummy' pill (an inactive compound – a 'placebo'). In addition, various classes of BP-lowering drugs have been compared against each other. There remain contentious areas, such as the debate about the superiority of one class of BP-lowering drug over another class, particularly in people with different risk profiles. It is likely that over the next 5 years more definitive answers about the relative effectiveness of different classes of BP-lowering drugs will become clearer. At present a large study in the US has recently shown that thiazide diuretics, one of the older classes of BP-lowering drugs, are as good as newer classes of BP-lowering drugs and should be regarded at the initial BP drug of choice for most people.

Is a thiazide diuretic the best drug to use? Hasn't this type been superseded by the newer classes of BP-lowering drugs?

Thiazide diuretics are probably the best studied class of BP-lowering drug. Thiazide diuretics decrease the rates of stroke and death. Low-dose thiazides are also associated with reduction in coronary heart disease. A recent landmark trial undertaken in the United States examined the relative effectiveness of four different classes of BP-lowering drugs – thiazide diuretic, ACE inhibitor, calcium-channel blocker and an alpha-adrenoceptor blocking drug. The study conclusively shows that thiazide diuretics produce identical results compared with calcium-channel blockers and ACE inhibitors in terms of a reduction of coronary heart disease, death and non-fatal heart attack. The centrally acting BP-lowering drug was shown to be inferior to the thiazide, particularly in those at risk from heart failure.

This US study is very reassuring. It is clear that thiazide diuretics will remain the mainstay of treatment for high BP for some time.

I am about to start on drugs for my high BP. What will I be given?

BP-lowering drugs are given according to the other risk factors that you may have. When you start a BP-lowering drug, your doctor should take into account your past medical history and risk factor profile when deciding on the most appropriate drug treatment. In addition you should be told about any side effects of the main classes of BP-lowering drugs. Appendix 1 gives a list of the contraindications and side effects of the most common drugs used to lower BP.

How do most people get on once they start taking a BP-lowering drug?

Recent studies of low-dose BP-lowering drugs have shown that they are well tolerated by most people. About three-quarters of people treated with any of the common class of BP-lowering drugs had remained on their drug treatment when they were followed up 4 years later. In drug comparison studies (comparison of different classes of BP-lowering drugs), all the different classes of drugs were tolerated equally well.

For most people thiazide diuretics remain the drugs of choice for those who have been newly diagnosed. The recent landmark study in the US has shown that they are safe, effective and cheap. They are as good (and in some circumstances) better than the newer BP-lowering drugs. So, your doctor will start you off on a thiazide diuretic but, if you have a particular risk profile, you might be started on a different BP-lowering drug. In general, alpha-antagonists and short-acting calcium-channel blockers are not given as a first drug.

You talk about side effects. What are the most common side effects of antihypertensive drugs and how frequently do they occur?

Tolerability and side effects are of course closely linked. However, side effects are specific to different classes of BP-lowering drug. Appendix 1 indicates the common side effects associated with each class. For example, about a quarter of people receiving calcium-channel blockers have reported ankle swelling, a third of people receiving an ACE inhibitor report a dry cough, and about 10% of people receiving beta-blockers report having cold hands and feet (but see also the question on asthma and beta-blockers in the section on *Problems requiring beta- or alpha-blockers* in Chapter 6). For most people, these side effects are not so disabling as to stop them taking their BP-lowering drug. However, if you experience a side effect, however trivial, it is always worth discussing this with your GP or practice nurse when you are being reviewed in your surgery or clinic. It is important to report these to your doctor, because they can nearly always be avoided by a change in drug or dose.

How do I go about finding what classes of BP-lowering drugs I am on?

To find out about your own medication, first look at the name printed by your chemist on the container. If you are on more than one drug, and you think that you are being treated for other problems as well as high BP, you must decide which of them is for your BP – if you're not sure, ask your chemist, or your doctor or practice nurse. Don't forget that drugs have both generic (scientific) names, and brand names. Generic names are used throughout this book and tend to be common internationally. Most people in the UK are now prescribed generic BP-lowering drugs. The table in Appendix 1 describes the common indications, contraindications and side effects of different classes of BP-lowering drugs.

I was told at my check-up that my prescription seemed to be working well. By how much is my BP likely to have been reduced?

Used on their own, BP-lowering drugs in current use usually reduce BP by about 5–15 mmHg diastolic and about 10–25 mmHg systolic pressure. This response is quite variable in individual people. If drugs from different groups are combined, their effects are usually additive: over two-thirds of people taking BP-lowering drugs finally require two or more different agents.

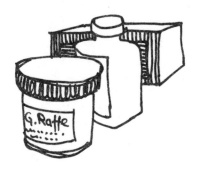

Taking your tablets

I have been on tablets for my high BP for over 2 years now. Will I ever be able to stop taking them?

Providing you are properly assessed initially and have sustained high BP, probably not. A few people rightly treated with definitely raised BP in their 30s seem to be able to stop taking medication after many years of good control, without returning to their original high pressure, but this seems to be rare. Even these people need careful supervision, with annual BP checks needed for the rest of their lives. Most people who stop medication have a gradual rise in BP, which often starts several months after stopping medication.

I am being changed onto slow-release tablets. What advantage will this have?

Slow-release (SR) tablets or capsules are designed to delay absorption in your stomach. SR preparations are much more expensive, more profitable, and are rarely available as 'generic' preparations, so manufacturers tend to promote them more energetically than is justified by their occasional real advantage.

Manufacturers claim that SR preparations help to supply drugs more evenly through the day, with consequent better control of BP. This is rarely important, because most of the drugs have a long half-life (which is the time taken for the blood level of a drug to fall to half its highest value), and so do their active metabolites (simpler but still usefully active chemicals resulting from chemical breakdown of the original drug). Manufacturers also claim that SR drugs give better control at night. As BP falls by as much as 10 to 50 mmHg during sleep, even in people with untreated severe high BP, this argument is rather unconvincing.

The real justification for SR preparations is in terms of avoiding unpleasant side effects at peak blood levels, or avoiding rebound high BP when blood levels fall. For these reasons, many calcium-channel blockers are best taken only as SR preparations.

My eating habits are a bit erratic. Should I take my SR tablets before, during or after meals?

All slow-release drugs are designed to be taken either with a meal, or soon after. Otherwise, timing in relation to meals is unimportant, except that a fixed routine is easier to remember.

I take another two types of tablets every day. Can I swallow my BP drugs at the same times as these other tablets for other problems?

Yes.

Because I take various other tablets, I am worried that my BP tablets might interact with these. Will it be safe to do this?

Diuretics are used to treat heart failure and swelling ('oedema') from kidney and heart problems, as well as for BP lowering. You have to watch out for this if you start taking ACE inhibitors because, if these are started simultaneously with diuretics, you may have a sudden very severe fall in BP, which can give you kidney failure. ACE inhibitors should be started on their own, although, once you have been taking them for some time, the doctor may add diuretics cautiously to increase their effect. People already on diuretics, who seem to need treatment with ACE inhibitors, may be referred to a hospital-based specialist, who may arrange for treatment to begin under close supervision in hospital. To make it more complicated, ACE inhibitors are also very effective for treating heart failure.

Otherwise the main potential interactions are with non-steroidal anti-inflammatory drugs (NSAIDs) used for treating arthritis and other bone, joint and muscular pains; with steroid drugs used to treat severe rheumatoid arthritis and asthma, and with some antidepressant drugs. These are all discussed in Chapter 6 and your doctor will be aware of any of these potential problems.

I rather like a drink in the evenings with my meal. Can I drink alcohol while on BP-lowering drugs?

Yes, within reason. No BP-lowering drugs have any specific harmful effects in combination with alcohol, but you must bear two things in mind.

- First, alcohol in excess of the recommended amounts

(more than 2 pints of beer, or 4 glasses of wine or single measures of spirits for a man of average size, a bit less for women – much less than social custom!) is itself an important cause of high BP. People who cannot get good control of their high BP despite normally adequate BP-lowering medication often find that, if they cut alcohol intake by half or more, they obtain good control with smaller doses of their drugs.

• Secondly, BP-lowering drugs that cause drowsiness (such as methyldopa,) will do so much more if combined with even small doses of alcohol. All other BP-lowering drugs cause some drowsiness in some people.

My memory isn't what it used to be! How can I remember to take my tablets?

The commonest problems are either forgetting completely, or wondering whether you actually took a tablet, a few minutes after taking it. Devise your own method, stick to it, and make sure that your partner knows it too, so that he or she can help you remember. Not taking your BP-lowering tablets is one of the main reasons why people fail to reach BP treatment goals. It is important to be honest with your GP as it is important to distinguish between people who are not responding to BP medication and require additional drugs and those who are not taking their tablets properly and have uncontrolled high BP for this reason.

Obviously, you should try to take your tablets always at the same times. Make sure that your doctor prescribes them to be taken once or twice a day, not three times. Shiftworkers can usually stick to the same times, if they are taking tablets only once or twice a day. Some branded tablets come in foil packs marked with the days of the week, like the contraceptive pill, and these are a great help. Your chemist will also be able to offer you a range of special containers designed to help you remember your medication – these are usually divided up into daily 'boxes' where you can place all your pills for the day.

If I do forget to take one of my tablets, what should I do?

Take your usual dose as soon as you remember it. **Don't** take a double dose, and don't worry about a couple of hours either way on dosage times.

So is taking a double dose dangerous?

This usually happens when people have just swallowed their tablets, but forget they have done so. That's why using a failsafe system is a good idea. None of the drugs used to lower BP is harmful in any important way if a single normal dose is doubled, although some of them could make you a bit drowsy.

What should I do if I can't swallow tablets because of a sore throat, or can't keep them down because of vomiting?

If you are ill enough not to be able to swallow or keep down tablets, you need to see your doctor, both for treatment and to have your BP checked.

Neither aspirin, paracetamol (called acetaminophen in the USA), antibiotics, nor any other medication likely to be bought or prescribed for sore throat, has any harmful interaction with BP-lowering drugs.

Some drugs used to treat nausea and vomiting (phenothiazines such as prochlorperazine [Stemetil]) can interact with methyldopa (Aldomet) to cause involuntary writhing movements of the face and limbs. This effect is reversible, won't last, and is not serious, but it can be very frightening. Metoclopramide (Maxolon) is an effective prescribed alternative. It also may cause involuntary movements of the same kind, particularly in children and young women, but does so more rarely. Otherwise you can buy hyoscine (Joyrides, Kwells, Scopoderm). These are less effective but do not have this side effect. Your illness is not likely to continue long enough for your BP to rise out of control.

When my BP has been controlled, can I stop taking the tablets altogether?

No. Your BP will probably rise to its pretreatment level, usually within a day or two, but occasionally up to 3 months after stopping.

BP-lowering drugs, mainly beta-blockers and calcium-channel blockers, also control angina. This also may transiently get much worse if you stop taking your drugs suddenly.

It seems sensible always to both start and stop BP-lowering drugs slowly, one step at a time, with BP checks between. You should be able to arrange these with your practice nurse or GP.

I sometimes feel very ill and I think it is because of my BP tablets. Can I vary the dose of my BP-lowering drugs according to how I feel from day to day?

Your symptoms are probably not related to BP except at very high and dangerous levels, which are rare. The only way to know about your BP reading is to measure it properly with a sphygmomanometer (see Chapter 3). The main value of home readings of BP using your own or a borrowed machine is that you will learn this from experience.

If you feel ill, you should consult your doctor or practice nurse. If you are convinced your medication is making you ill, stop taking it, and see your doctor as soon as possible.

I am about to go into hospital for an operation. What should I do about taking my BP drugs when I'm there?

The most sensible policy is usually to take with you just enough of your tablets to last a day or two, putting them in envelopes with their names and strength written on the outside.

Most admissions are for planned surgery, when the only doctor likely to show much interest in high BP is the anaesthetist. Most hospitals allow people to continue their medication, but may still insist on supplying their own drugs during your stay in hospital.

I know I leave my tablets lying around sometimes. Are BP-lowering drugs dangerous if taken accidentally or misused?

None of the drugs commonly used for high BP is much good for killing either yourself or others! All are widely tolerated between the lowest and highest effective doses, and there is a large margin between the highest effective dose and a lethal dose. Some are dangerous to children and, for this reason, **all** drugs should be locked out of harm's way.

I ran short of my BP drugs the other week before I could get my repeat prescription. If this happens again, can I borrow some from my friend, who is also being treated for high BP?

No – this is not to be recommended and should only be done in an emergency; even then, you should do this only if you are completely certain that your friend's tablets are identical to your own. Check both the name and the strength on the chemist's label, and look carefully at the tablets themselves.

If there is the slightest doubt about this, **do not take chances**. Although there is little difference in effectiveness or tolerability between the large number of different tablets available, they work in different ways, and it is very unwise to start mixing up treatments yourself.

Keep an eye on how many tablets you have left, and make sure that you get a repeat prescription well before they run out. Trying to get prescriptions at weekends can be difficult, so plan ahead.

6
High blood pressure with other problems

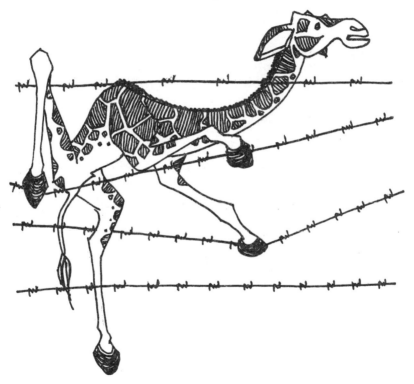

High blood pressure is rarely a singular condition. More often high BP occurs in conjunction with other medical conditions. These conditions can alter a person's risk of stroke or heart attack (cardiovascular disease) or require 'tailoring' of BP drugs. Heart problems, diabetes and kidney disease are all conditions that are associated with increased risk of such problems and, if

BP is raised as well, doctors will start you on BP-lowering drugs with a target level in mind. Other conditions discussed in this chapter are not associated in themselves with increased risk but have important implications in terms of selecting the right drug for you.

Heart problems

I know that I am overweight and am having difficulty in giving up smoking. You have spoken about risk factors that might increase my chances of having a stroke or heart attack. How will all this relate to what drugs are chosen for reducing my BP?

Assessment of your risk is necessary in order to choose the right drugs for you and your specific circumstances. Absolute risk assessment seeks to identify all important risk factors that may need treatment as well as high BP. It can also establish the absolute benefit each person can expect from particular drug and non-drug treatments. For some people, there may be other risks that take precedence over the treatment of high BP. For example, someone with bad chronic obstructive airways disease and urinary incontinence has more immediate problems in terms of quality of life and alleviation of discomfort than the introduction of another set of drugs, which may make management of their obstructive airways disease and urinary incontinence worse.

Prioritization of treatments for people like yourself with perhaps multiple cardiovascular risk factors and coexisting conditions is very difficult both for health professionals and for the people themselves. Making decisions about which risks take precedence and how treatment should be tailored to address these is a time-consuming and challenging process. Information about different risks is now becoming increasingly available in the media. When making a decision about various treatments, you need to consider the expected benefits and harms, the interaction of drug treatment for high BP with any other conditions that you might have, and what your own personal value and preferences about life-long treatment might be.

I have been diagnosed with angina and now to top it all I have high BP as well. What drugs are likely to help me the most?

People with angina or who have suffered a heart attack ('myocardial infarction') are by definition at high risk of suffering another attack. In people with a history of angina, and particularly in those who have had a previous heart attack, beta-blockers have been shown to have clear benefits in both relief of symptoms of angina and reduced risk of death from heart attacks. For this reason beta-blockers are often used as the first treatment for high BP. Calcium-channel blockers may also provide symptomatic relief for angina. ACE inhibitor drugs have been shown to be highly effective in reducing mortality, particularly if you have a high risk of cardiovascular disease. In people with a history of heart attack, who also suffer from heart failure, calcium-channel blockers are not recommended.

I suffered a heart attack recently and have now developed heart failure. What drugs are most effective for my raised BP and what drugs should I avoid?

In people with heart failure, ACE inhibitors are the best treatment. They have been shown to reduce the risk of death irrespective of heart failure severity.

Angiotensin II receptor blockers have also been shown to be highly effective in people with heart failure. These are generally reserved as second-line drugs in people in whom side effects of ACE inhibitors are troublesome or in whom symptoms of heart failure are not sufficiently relieved. Beta-blockers also are good for heart failure and can be recommended for BP lowering with additional benefits in people with heart failure.

Alpha-adrenoceptor blocking drugs and long-acting calcium-channel blockers are associated with worsening of heart failure and increasing risk of death.

I have an irregular heartbeat, which my doctor says is caused by what they called 'atrial fibrillation'. What is this exactly and how does it affect management of my high BP?

Atrial fibrillation means irregular and uncoordinated movement of the fibres of heart muscle, so that, instead of acting effectively together to squeeze blood through the heart, they form an ineffective, trembling bag. When this happens in the main chambers of the heart, the 'ventricles', your heart stops and you die unless someone can stop this process by giving your heart an electric shock. Atrial fibrillation affects only the two upper and less important chambers of the heart, the auricles or atria.

Atrial fibrillation is quite common, particularly in people aged over 70. Occasionally, normal heart rhythm can be restored, either by drugs or by giving a controlled electric shock, sometimes followed by insertion of a pacemaker to maintain normal rhythm. This is rarely necessary. The most important issue is to prevent blood clots forming in the atrial chambers of your heart by using anticoagulants such as warfarin or aspirin. Thinning of the blood has been shown to prevent the clots in the atria becoming dislodged, travelling to your brain and causing a stroke. If you do have atrial fibrillation, it is important that you consider taking some form of blood-thinning drug to reduce your risk. Your risk of suffering a stroke will be determined by your age (your risk of stroke increases as you get older), whether or not you have suffered a stroke or a mini-stroke ('transient ischaemic attack' or TIA) in the past, whether you suffer from heart failure or whether you suffer from high blood pressure.

Many people who suffer from heart failure also suffer from atrial fibrillation. For most people with heart failure, treatment with ACE inhibitors, diuretics, and sometimes digoxin, to slow their heart rate and raise heart output, alleviates symptoms and improves their quality of life. They usually take some form of blood-thinning medication as well, to reduce their risk of stroke.

If you also have high BP, this is likely to have been one of the main causes of your heart failure. Paradoxically, your BP will tend to fall as your heart fails, and to rise as heart failure is controlled and heart output rises. The main consequence for management is that you will need carefully balanced medication, both to treat your heart failure, to make sure your BP doesn't go too high again, and to control the thinness of your blood. Your kidney and liver functions will be monitored closely by regular blood tests.

I am aged 70. Will I be offered anything different for my raised BP because of my age?

Older people (those aged over 65 years) have a greater risk of stroke or heart attack because of their age alone. Low-dose diuretics have been shown to be highly effective for older people with high BP. An alternative is a calcium-channel blocker if you can't be given thiazides. Rather confusingly, a recent large scale clinical trial in the USA compared a thiazide diuretic to an ACE inhibitor. The ACE inhibitor was superior to the thiazide in reducing combined cardiovascular (stroke and heart attack) risks, despite a similar degree of BP lowering. At present there is some confusion about which class of BP-lowering drug is the best for initial treatment in older people. Current opinion is that attention should be focused on good BP control, irrespective of which agent – thiazide, calcium-channel blocker or ACE inhibitor – is used.

Calcium-channel blockers would not normally be given if you have already had a heart attack. Side effects of all drugs are given in Appendix 1.

Diabetes

I have had diabetes for some years. I understand I'm at greater risk of suffering a stroke or heart attack. What are the recommended treatments for somebody with diabetes and high BP?

Mortality from cardiovascular disease is increased two- or three-fold in people with both hypertension and diabetes compared to those in the general population. For this reason, the combination of diabetes and hypertension has been labelled as 'double jeopardy'. There have been many studies that have shown that ACE inhibitors, beta-blockers and low-dose thiazide diuretics are effective in reducing this risk of dying from a heart attack or stroke.

If you have diabetes and high BP you will be seen as having combined risk factors and you will be told that control of your blood sugar and BP levels is very important. Your treatment will be intensified so that you reach your target BP, cholesterol and blood sugar levels. Studies have shown that treatment should be aimed at lowering BP to below 130/80 mmHg, total cholesterol to less than 5 mmol/litre and glycosylated haemoglobin (long-acting sugar level indicator) to below 5%.

Whether an ACE inhibitor, beta-blocker or low-dose thiazide diuretic is used in the treatment of your raised BP alongside your diabetes is not important. These drugs have produced equivalent results in clinical studies.

Kidney problems

I have had some kidney problems recently and I am worried about now having to be treated for raised BP. What will I be given?

ACE inhibitors and angiotensin II receptor blockers have been shown to reduce death from and progression of kidney disease, so these drugs will be the preferred ones for people like yourself with raised BP and kidney problems. People with diabetes (see question above) tend to suffer from kidney problems as an additional complication of their diabetes, so many are treated with ACE inhibitors, as these are more effective in helping to slow down the progression of kidney disease.

I have been told that I have chronic renal failure. What does this mean? I was also told that I am very likely to need BP-lowering drugs. Why, and what are they doing?

Chronic kidney ('renal') disease can be classified as being due to a diminished excretory function (improperly filtering toxic waste products from the blood) or leakage of protein from the kidney in the urine. Both forms often occur together. High BP often occurs following these types of kidney problems, because the kidney has a critical role in maintaining blood volume by means of the renin–angiotensin system (see Chapter 2). The commonest reason for chronic renal failure is as a result of diabetes (see previous section), but other causes of chronic renal failure do occur.

If blood pressure remains high, end-stage renal disease will follow more swiftly, which requires dialysis. In addition, chronic renal disease also increases your risk of heart attack and stroke. BP treatment has two important benefits. Firstly, it helps to slow down renal failure, reducing the risk of end-stage renal failure and dialysis. Secondly, overall cardiovascular risk is reduced.

To get these benefits, good BP control, often with three or more drugs to reach target BP levels, is required. Paradoxically, treatment with ACE inhibitors and ACE II receptor blockers may cause mild kidney problems. This means that you might be referred to a specialist, if you have chronic kidney disease, for appropriate monitoring of your renal function and tailoring of drug treatment.

Raised cholesterol levels

I have had a lipid test recently and my cholesterol levels were found to be on the high side. Will this be a problem in my treatment for high BP?

Lipid level abnormalities are often present in people with high BP. They both contribute to an increased risk of cardiovascular disease. Dietary changes in people with raised plasma cholesterol is discussed in Chapter 4.

Evidence now suggests that the BP-lowering effects of such drugs as diuretics and beta-blockers exceed any possible changes in people's lipid profiles. Therefore, even in people with raised cholesterol levels, treatment with thiazides and beta-blockers can still be recommended as a first treatment.

What will I probably be given?

Statins are very effective in reducing LDL and VLDL blood cholesterol (see Chapter 4 for an explanation of these terms). Inflammation of muscle cells ('myositis') has occurred in about 1 in 200 people treated, causing muscle pain, weakness or unexplained fever. Other possible side effects are headache and liver damage. Regular monitoring of liver function is recommended, every 6 weeks for the first 15 months and occasionally thereafter.

Statins are a new class of very effective and well tolerated cholesterol-lowering drugs, introduced in 1989. So far there are five drugs in this group, pravastatin (Lipostat), atorvastatin (Lipitor), cerivastatin (Lipobay), fluvastatin (Lescol) and simvastatin (Zocor). They act by inhibiting an enzyme involved in cholesterol synthesis.

It has been shown that statins are highly effective drugs for people both with and without existing coronary heart disease. Recent randomized trials of statins in patients with high BP (who hadn't suffered a heart attack in the past) have shown that the chance of suffering a fatal or non-fatal heart attack was reduced from 5% to 3% over 5 years. In women, at lower such risk, the benefits of statins may well be more modest. Current thinking is that people with moderately raised cholesterol levels should have their risk assessed, and that their BP and cholesterol treatment should be decided in the light of this assessment.

Problems requiring beta- or alpha-blockers

I have severe asthma and my doctor would not put me on beta-blockers for my raised BP. Why should these drugs be avoided in people with asthma?

Beta-blockers increase airways obstruction in people with recognized or latent asthma. However, as beta-blockers have different effects on the airways (known as 'selective' or 'non-selective beta-blockers'), some types of beta-blockers are more harmful than others. Some people with chronic bronchitis or emphysema also have unrecognized asthma. There have been deaths from using beta-blockers in these people, so before starting beta-blockers, the doctor will measure airways resistance in anyone with any kind of bad chest. More often than not, there are alternative BP-lowering agents that can be used in these situations. Generally speaking selective beta-blocker agents, i.e. drugs that act only on the heart rather than on the lung airways, are preferred to non-selective agents. Non-selective beta-blockers must be avoided in people with asthma or obstructive airways disease. Selective beta-blockers can be used in certain circumstances where alternative BP-lowering drugs are not available or where obstructive airways disease can only be improved slightly.

I suffer from migraine every month. I have now been diagnosed with high BP. Will this affect which drugs I am prescribed?

Beta-blockers are used to prevent the onset of migrainous headache. For this reason they are generally preferred for people who suffer from migraines and high BP, so you will probably be offered these first to see how you get on.

I have been given beta-blockers for my high BP and found later that I had real problems making love to my wife. Would it have been the drugs that were causing my erection problems? Could I be given something else for the BP?

You are quite correct. Beta-blockers are associated with erection problems but to a lesser extent than diuretics. As many as 15–20% of men taking high dose diuretics (e.g. 5 mg bendrofluazide) experience it. If you are having problems in this department, do go to your doctor and discuss them because there will be other drugs that you could be prescribed instead. Sexual dysfunction is discussed in more detail in Chapter 8.

I suffer from prostatic symptoms. Are there some BP-lowering drugs more suitable for me?

Alpha-adrenoceptor blocking drugs have the effect of reducing BP and simultaneously relieving symptoms of prostate obstruction. However, trials of alpha-blockers have not been good, apparently increasing risk of heart failure. They are not given if you suffer from heart failure. Your doctor will be able to discuss what other types of drugs are available.

Blood-thinning drugs

I have been told to take a small dose of aspirin every day, but I also take high BP drugs for my BP. Are there any risks of taking aspirin when I have high BP as well?

Aspirin is a drug that has substantial benefits – mostly by reducing your risk of stroke and heart attack – but is also associated with side effects, usually by causing bleeding in your stomach. People at high risk of a stroke or heart attack (usually taken to be over 5% over 5 years) generally gain substantially more benefit than harm from aspirin. If you are taking non-steroidal anti-inflammatory drugs, your risk of suffering such bleeding will be increased further, so these should be avoided if possible. Talk to your doctor about your concerns – you should always alert the doctor to the fact that you are taking other drugs when the question of treatment for high BP is being discussed. You may be talking to a different doctor than usual and so he or she may be unaware of your other problems.

Anticoagulants such as warfarin or heparin are prescribed almost always by specialists. You can't avoid taking them then, but those who do prescribe them will always review your need for aspirin.

Racial differences

My family came from Jamaica originally and my father has high BP. It seems to run in our family. Do black people differ from white people in the way that they respond to BP-lowering drugs?

African-Caribbean black people are at particular risk of developing high BP. High BP also tends to be more severe, with a higher risk of complications, particularly stroke and renal failure. Non-drug treatment, particularly cutting down on salt, seems to be more effective in this group of people.

As regards drug treatment, yes, people from African-Caribbean descent respond less well to beta-blocker drugs and to ACE inhibitors, related to the fact that the renin–angiotensin system is suppressed in this group (see Chapter 2). It has been shown that they respond better than other ethnic groups to thiazide diuretics and calcium-channel blockers.

Similarly, people with a southern Asian background have a higher chance of developing high BP and diabetes, being particularly at risk of developing coronary heart disease. However, their response to BP-lowering drugs is similar to that of people from white European descent. Asian people need to be particularly careful about their coronary heart disease risk and often benefit from aspirin and statin treatment as well as their BP medication.

Pain – particularly joint pain and arthritis

I've got to go on to tablets for high BP but also have arthritis and take ibuprofen for the pain. Will my treatment for arthritis affect what I am given for high BP?

Joint pains generally arise from osteoarthritis or inflammatory arthritis – most commonly rheumatoid arthritis, or gout. Treatment is usually with a non-steroidal anti-inflammatory drug (NSAID). There are many of these drugs, with some – such as ibuprofen (Brufen, Fenbid) – now available across the counter at chemists.

All the NSAIDs are usually effective for treatment of inflammatory arthritis and gout. Their effect on acute gout is usually dramatic. They can help people with osteoarthritis but their effect is usually less dramatic. They are also used in the treatment of period pains and heavy menstrual blood loss ('menorrhagia'), and mefenamic acid (Ponstan) has been particularly promoted for this.

Most NSAIDs raise BP by an average of 5–6 mmHg diastolic pressure, roughly the same as the reduction produced by most BP-lowering drugs. They appear to cause salt retention. Approximately, 40% of all people needing BP-lowering drugs also suffer from chronic rheumatic pains and NSAIDs are often given. You need to be aware of the effect of NSAIDs on your BP and ask your doctor for alternative treatment – paracetamol, which is not an NSAID, can provide very effective pain relief without any of the side effects on BP increase. Ibuprofen, which is available over the counter, has a much smaller effect than most other NSAIDs, averaging less than 2 mmHg. You should ask a pharmacist if the drug you are buying is likely to affect your BP or interact with your BP-lowering drugs.

I have severe rheumatoid arthritis treated with steroid tablets (prednisolone). Will this affect my treatment for high BP?

Steroid drugs (usually in the form of prednisone or adrencortico-trophic hormone – ACTH) are necessary and effective for severe, acute attacks of rheumatoid arthritis, particularly in the first few months after onset of the disease. In these circumstances they may not only relieve pain, but also reduce long-term joint damage. Although they raise BP by causing salt and water retention, and thus increasing blood volume, this is almost always a price worth paying, even for people with severe high BP. In any case, these severe cases will usually be under the care of a hospital specialist, whose job it is to make a balanced decision in the light of all the evidence of your particular case.

Long-term use of steroids for rheumatoid arthritis not only raises BP (seldom by very much), but weakens bone structure with a high risk of spontaneous fractures of the spine, which reduces breathing capacity and resistance to infections of all kinds. There are alternative disease-modifying drugs that are available and you can ask your GP or specialist about them. Rheumatologists normally keep people with rheumatoid arthritis off steroids for as long as possible. Raised BP, even in people with high BP, is one of the smaller risks of long-term steroids.

I have had several attacks of gout in the past and I am now on BP-lowering drugs. I have been told certain types of BP-lowering drugs can cause gout. Is this true?

Gout occurs when your body fails to get rid of one of its waste products, a substance called uric acid. Usually the kidneys get rid of the uric acid in your blood, and it is passed out in your urine. In you develop gout, you have a metabolic disturbance and too much uric acid is produced and accumulates as crystals in the joints of your body. This can result in severe pain, swelling, redness and tenderness of the affected joint, most often your big toe joint. It is a common problem and does tend to run in families.

Uric acid levels in your blood can be raised by alcohol, some foods (liver is a good example) and by thiazide diuretics in high dosage. At low dosage (usually 2.5 mg bendrofluazide daily), there is rarely any effect on uric acid levels, and at 1.25 mg there is no effect at all. These low doses are just as effective in controlling BP. Gout was a particular problem in people taking high-dose thiazides but, as the BP-lowering benefits can be achieved with low-dose thiazides, the side effect of gout is much less common.

There is some evidence that, in people who have a tendency towards suffering gout (past history or family history),higher dosage thiazide diuretics double the risk of suffering a recurrence of gout. So thiazide diuretics will not be given to you – alternative BP-lowering drugs will be prescribed.

Psychological problems

My mother has developed schizophrenia but she also has high BP. Will her condition affect what she is prescribed for hypertension?

Most people with schizophrenia are treated permanently with major tranquillizer drugs – the phenothiazines – either as tablets or depot injections once a month. These drugs have a powerful BP-lowering effect, which usually makes any other BP-lowering medication unnecessary.

Involuntary writhing movements, usually of the face and limbs, are a common complication of long-term treatment with phenothiazines. This effect is increased by methyldopa (Aldomet), which should therefore not be used to treat high BP in schizophrenics.

7
Pregnancy, contraception and the menopause

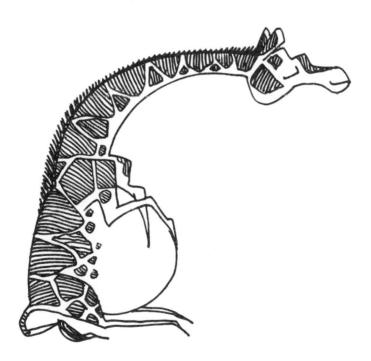

This chapter covers the issue of high blood pressure in pregnancy, discussing the related issues of planning a pregnancy, monitoring of BP during pregnancy and management of delivery in the light of having high BP during pregnancy. Contraception and hormone replacement therapy (HRT) are also discussed.

High BP and planning a pregnancy

I have had high BP for several years and would now like to plan a pregnancy. What precautions should I take?

The most sensible approach for a woman with known high BP planning a pregnancy is to seek prepregnancy advice from a well-informed GP, physician or specialist obstetrician. General advice will include maintaining a sensible balanced diet and normal weight for your height, taking regular exercise, stopping smoking and either stopping alcohol or keeping intake to a minimum. All women who are planning a pregnancy are advised to take extra folic acid (a vitamin that plays an important part in the development of the fetus) for 3 months before a planned pregnancy (e.g. before you stop using contraceptives) and for the first 3 months of pregnancy. Specific advice will relate to whether your high BP requires treatment, what BP-lowering drugs are safe to use in pregnancy, whether you could stop your medication for the early part of pregnancy and whether there are additional risks to your health or that of your baby because of your high BP. It is highly unlikely that you will be advised not to have a pregnancy because of high BP.

We hear a lot about how drugs taken in pregnancy can damage unborn babies – I'm especially thinking of thalidomide, but I know there are others. Can BP-lowering drugs be safely taken in pregnancy?

The time when we are most concerned about drugs affecting the fetus (the unborn baby) is in early pregnancy. Your pregnancy begins before you miss your period, but for the first week when the fertilized egg is moving down your fallopian tube, it is probably not at risk from drugs in your bloodstream. The important time for development is from the time of implantation up until the end of the third month, a period known as 'organogenesis' because all of the baby's organs and structures are developing. After the first 3 months of pregnancy the baby is mostly just growing and is much less vulnerable to any effects from drugs.

If you are taking BP-lowering drugs, then you should take the earliest opportunity to discuss with your GP (or whoever else is looking after your BP) whether or not you need to change your type of drug or whether it would be safe for you to stop treatment. Ideally this will have been planned before your pregnancy as discussed in the previous question.

Ever since thalidomide (which, incidentally, was a sleeping tablet and was used for morning sickness – it was not a BP-lowering drug), all drugs have been tested on animals (mostly rabbits or rats) to see if they might cause organ damage to the fetus during pregnancy. Because very large numbers of animals can be used, these tests are fairly sensitive, but because they are not on humans, we can never be entirely sure that they exclude risks to a human fetus. New drugs are rarely tested in pregnant women and often not even in women of reproductive age. We have to rely on more indirect evidence from population-based studies and on reporting of bad outcomes (adverse event reporting) where pregnant women have inadvertently taken drugs.

Thousands of women and babies have been checked in this way for evidence of fetal damage from drugs taken in pregnancy and, on the whole, these studies have been reassuring. None of the common BP-lowering drugs has been shown to produce fetal damage, although many women have conceived while taking their regular BP-lowering medication. Unfortunately this is not the same as proving safety. Although damage on the scale of thalidomide is certainly not happening, serious damage to as few as 1 baby in every 1000 born is possible. We have to take this risk seriously, while at the same time not being alarmist. Naturally there is greatest experience and reassurance about safety with the older BP-lowering drugs. For this reason, you may be advised to change from a newer type of BP-lowering drug to a more old-fashioned one when planning a pregnancy or when you are seen in the early stages of an unplanned pregnancy.

What does this mean in practice? There are three things to consider.

- BP-lowering drugs should be avoided in pregnancy, unless your raised BP is serious enough to justify this.

- Plan your pregnancies with the help of a well informed GP or obstetrician and, if you do need BP-lowering drugs, you can be confident that you will be prescribed the safest possible choice.

- Discuss the possibility of temporarily interrupting your treatment with BP-lowering drugs during the weeks when you are attempting to conceive and during the first 13 weeks of your pregnancy.

I have tried different BP-lowering drugs for my hypertension and they haven't always suited me. What options will I have in pregnancy?

You will obviously want to avoid any drugs that could cause additional risk to you or to your baby. Methyldopa is an old-fashioned drug, which, although it does have some side effects, has a good track record for safety and effectiveness at all stages of pregnancy.

Beta-blockers are well tolerated and apparently without risk to the baby after 24 weeks; before this they may slow down the baby's growth and should be given only if necessary. There is most experience with labetalol, but atenolol should be avoided as this agent was implicated in a small study showing impaired growth in fetuses.

The calcium-channel blockers are commonly used in later pregnancy, but there is much less safety data than for methyldopa or beta-blockers and they are best avoided in early pregnancy unless there are reasons for not being prescribed other types.

Diuretics, often the first choice for high BP, are ruled out because they may make pre-eclampsia worse (pre-eclampsia is discussed later in this chapter). However, this risk is probably theoretical and many women will have taken diuretics in early pregnancy with little evidence of side effects to themselves or their babies. However, you will probably not be given them in pregnancy.

The drugs that really need to be avoided for your baby's sake are the ACE inhibitors, which have known dangers for the developing baby (usually later in pregnancy) and newer agents that are completely unevaluated in pregnancy. As you will see from Appendix 1 (where there is more information about all these drugs), that still leaves you and your doctor with plenty of choices.

High BP in pregnancy

I have heard that BP falls in pregnancy. Why is this?

Yes, it normally falls during pregnancy. This is one of the reasons why you may be able to stop BP-lowering drugs for at least part of your pregnancy. If it rises, this is always important, because it may indicate that you have pre-eclampsia or eclampsia (the next section in this chapter deals with both these conditions). Nurses, doctors, and midwives regularly measure your BP all through pregnancy looking for newly elevated BP or the development of pre-eclampsia.

Pregnancy normally lasts between 38 and 42 weeks. This is usually divided into three periods of development, called trimesters. The first 13 weeks (the first trimester) roughly corresponds to the time when the baby is being formed. The second trimester is from 14 to 27 weeks: it used to be the time when the baby was thought to be too immature to survive, but now some babies as young as 24 weeks do survive with intensive neonatal care. Babies were considered able to survive if they were born during the third trimester (which runs from 28 weeks of pregnancy until the birth), although before modern intensive care many failed to do so.

From whatever level it starts, your BP normally falls during the second trimester (from 14 to 27 weeks). It then usually rises slowly until your baby is born (which is normally at 38 to 42 weeks), although it may still be a bit lower than before you became pregnant. After your baby is born your BP rises slowly over the first 5 days to regain its usual level before your pregnancy.

When you are pregnant, not only do you need oxygen, but so does your developing baby. Your body therefore makes more blood to carry enough oxygen for both of you, so the total volume of your blood rises rapidly during the first 12 to 13 weeks of your pregnancy. All other things being equal, a rise in blood volume should cause a rise in BP. To prevent this, your placenta (which nourishes your baby in your womb, links your blood supply with your baby's, and is expelled in the afterbirth following the birth of your baby) releases hormones (mainly progesterone), which relax the walls of your veins and small arteries so that they become larger to make room for this increased blood volume, without any rise in your BP. Because of this, your heart doesn't have to pump so hard and your BP falls.

Because your blood vessels are relaxed, they do not respond as quickly to instructions from your brain, so blood may remain in your legs when you get up out of a chair. Your BP then falls, and you may feel dizzy or faint. All this usually happens in the first 12 weeks or so when your circulation is changing most rapidly, but even later in pregnancy you may find yourself feeling faint in a hot room or if you get up too quickly from lying down. If this happens you should either sit or lie down and it will usually pass off quite quickly.

When I'm pregnant, how high must my BP be to be called high BP?

A BP of 140/90 mmHg or more is conventionally considered to be a high BP in pregnancy. The significance of these figures will depend on whether your high BP is new (i.e. developing for the first time in your pregnancy) or whether it was already high before you became pregnant.

Why is it important to know if my raised BP developed before I became pregnant or whether it is something new?

The difference between pregnancy in women with pre-existing high BP (i.e. having raised BP before you became pregnant) and high BP starting in pregnancy is simply the rate of change of your BP. Pre-existing high BP starts very slowly, in childhood or adolescence, with plenty of time for every part of your body to get used to it. High BP developing for the first time during pregnancy develops over a very short time, never more than a few weeks and occasionally even over a few hours. During this time you may get very serious damage to your small arteries, particularly in the kidneys, liver and brain. It may also affect the blood supply to the placenta and ultimately the oxygen supply to your unborn baby. The same kinds of damage may occur in pre-existing high BP, but only at much higher levels of BP, and usually over much longer periods of time.

If I get high BP during my pregnancy, who should look after it, my GP or my obstetrician?

If your BP rises for the first time during pregnancy, i.e. you didn't have high BP before you were pregnant, then your obstetrician will take the decisions about your treatment, although your GP and midwife also need to know what drugs (if any) you are taking. Because BP can change very quickly in pregnancy, your GP or midwife should check your BP if at any time you feel ill, have pain in the upper part of your abdomen, or a prolonged headache. These are important warning signs of pre-eclampsia (see next section). Your antenatal clinic should give you your maternity notes so that you can show them to anyone you need to consult, although in some areas you may instead be given a card called a shared-care card on which all this information can be recorded. Don't forget to take your notes with you whenever you go to the clinic or to see your GP.

Not many women are both young enough to be pregnant and at the same time old enough to have BP high enough to need BP-lowering medication. This means that not many obstetricians see women with long-standing high BP who have already had treatment for months or years. However, this pattern is changing with more women delaying child bearing to an older age, and you may well have a choice of healthcare professionals who can offer care. If you are affected by high BP, then you need joint care, intelligently shared between your GP or your hospital physician, your obstetrician and your midwife. Because your medication is likely to be changed during your pregnancy, you will need more frequent BP measurements than most women, and they will need to be very accurate.

I'm in my first pregnancy, and my BP has gone up a bit. My doctor says she'll keep an eye on it but that I don't need any drugs for it yet. If I do need to take BP-lowering drugs, when will I start on them?

Speaking generally, if BP rises for the first time after 36 weeks of pregnancy, then it is usually best to deliver the baby within a reasonable interval, so labour is brought on early (induced). This decision may be made without you needing BP-lowering drugs. If BP starts rising for the first time between 24 and 30 weeks, doctors usually try to control it with BP-lowering drugs so that the baby is more mature when born and has a better chance of surviving. Between 30 and 36 weeks BP-lowering drugs may help to prolong the pregnancy and increase the likelihood of you being able to have a normal delivery and reduce the likelihood of the baby needing medical support in the intensive care unit.

Doctors vary in their opinions on how high your BP should be before you start treatment. There is good evidence that treatment benefits both mother and baby when systolic BP measures 170 mmHg or more or diastolic BP measures 110 mmHg or more. This level of high BP is an indication for admission to hospital and immediate stabilization on BP-lowering drugs. There is far greater variation in practice when BP is between 140/90 and 160/100, what is called mild to moderate hypertension. Some studies suggest that treatment of mild to moderate hypertension may reduce the chance of progression to severe hypertension; however, the counter argument is that there may be a negative effect on the growth of the baby. There is clearly a balance to be achieved in treating moderate hypertension in pregnancy between potential benefit and harm. You will need to discuss this with your obstetrician who can take account of your individual circumstances and what approach is likely to result in the best outcome for you and your baby.

Pre-eclampsia and eclampsia

Could you explain what pre-eclampsia is?

Pre-eclampsia is a complication of pregnancy characterized by high BP, protein in the urine and oedema (swelling). These features do not always present at the same time, which can make the diagnosis difficult. The early stages are often symptomless and detection relies, therefore, on regular antenatal checks of your BP and urine. The majority of women who develop pre-eclampsia will develop only a mild form and will recover well with delivery of a healthy baby. However, it is potentially life-threatening to you and your baby if it is allowed to develop and progress without detection or appropriate management. Mothers with pre-eclampsia can be stabilized but it is only curable by delivery, which puts some babies at risk of death or disability from prematurity.

We do know that, as with pre-existing high BP, there is an inherited tendency for pre-eclampsia to run in families, which is why midwives and doctors ask you about BP in your relatives, particularly in your mother or sisters. Pre-eclampsia is also more common in first pregnancies, in women over 40, and in women who already have raised BP before they get pregnant. Your risk of pre-eclampsia is usually assessed at this first antenatal visit and the appropriate pattern of antenatal care will be determined at that time. Visits will be increased if complications are identified as your pregnancy progresses.

I'm worried that I may get pre-eclampsia when I get pregnant as I already have high BP. Am I at greater risk than women who don't already have high BP?

Pre-eclampsia is a condition in pregnancy that usually presents with high BP, protein in the urine and swelling (oedema). Your risk of pre-eclampsia is higher if you already have high BP but we don't know by exactly how much. Depending on your age, weight and family history, your risk of pre-eclampsia can be anything from 2 to 10 times that of a woman who did not have raised BP at the beginning of her pregnancy.

The problem is that, because most studies have been based on women attending hospital antenatal clinics, they often lack information about BP in women before their pregnancies began. If women are not seen for antenatal care until they are well into their pregnancies at 15–20 weeks (which is still fairly common in women at the highest risk of pre-eclampsia), and if there are no previous medical records about BP, then there is simply no way of knowing whether a rather high BP is recent and important, or it is long-standing and therefore much less important. A lot of research on this subject has been weakened by this lack of information, so any conclusions have to remain rather uncertain.

The moral of this is that, if any doctor or nurse has at any time been concerned about your BP, you should make sure the details of this are available to whichever professionals become responsible for advising you during your pregnancy. This information will influence your subsequent risk of pre-eclampsia and how your antenatal care is planned.

Because I suffered from pre-eclampsia in my first pregnancy, I have been looking up the subject now that I am pregnant again. I have see the words 'fulminating pre-eclampsia', which sounds very daunting. What is fulminating pre-eclampsia?

Fulminating is yet another word that comes from the Latin, and roughly means 'like lightning'. It can be applied to any illness or condition (not just pre-eclampsia) when it occurs suddenly and with great intensity (in other words, one which strikes like lightning).

Fulminating pre-eclampsia happens very rarely, but when it does, it is an emergency. The term is used to describe the extremely rapid development of pre-eclampsia, over hours or days rather than the more usual weeks. In this rare emergency, BP rises rapidly, large and increasing amounts of protein are passed in urine and fluid is retained so that the face swells up visibly over a few hours. When this happens the brain can also becomes swollen, and there is then immediate danger of eclamptic fits. Drugs will be used to bring down BP and to prevent fits (usually given by a drip in a vein), and the baby will be delivered as soon as possible either by inducing labour or by caesarean section. Recent research has shown that the best available treatment for women who develop an eclamptic fit is with magnesium (Epsom salts) given into a vein or into a muscle. This hospital treatment decreases the risk of further fits and reduces the danger to both mother and baby.

I presume 'pre-eclampsia' just means 'before eclampsia', but what exactly is eclampsia?

The word eclampsia comes from the Latin, and literally means 'flashing lights'. In practice it means fits (seizures) caused by brain damage, caused in turn by very high BP that develops very fast, usually in late pregnancy. Women suffering eclampsia usually see flashing lights just before a fit begins, hence the name. Soon after this, the sufferer suddenly loses consciousness, her whole body shakes symmetrically and uncontrollably, with clenched teeth and severe spasm of all muscles, all for only a minute or two but seeming much longer.

Eclampsia is very dangerous both to the mother and to the unborn child. Before modern antenatal care, deaths from eclampsia in pregnancy were common. They still happen, although very rarely – only in 10 pregnancies in every million.

In nearly all cases eclampsia is preceded by pre-eclampsia – either by several weeks of slowly rising BP, or by dramatic warning signs (mainly pain in the upper abdomen caused by congestion of the liver), or by severe persistent headache. The existence of these changes and warning signs means that nearly all cases of eclampsia can be prevented by good antenatal care. Because pregnancy is now normally well supervised, eclampsia has become very rare and, when it occurs, it may indicate a serious breakdown in health care.

Eclampsia is treated by urgent admission to hospital, by giving drugs to control BP and seizures, and by delivering the baby as quickly as possible, after which BP usually falls rapidly to normal without any other treatment.

Does anyone know what causes pre-eclampsia and eclampsia?

Although eclampsia was first identified 150 years ago, its prime cause remains unknown. When we do understand the cause we shall probably find that we should actually be talking about causes in the plural. We already know that there are different patterns to pre-eclampsia, and that these are likely to have different underlying causes.

Pre-eclampsia is somehow related to the placenta. The placenta has its own arteries. In pre-eclampsia these arteries do not penetrate the wall of the uterus (womb) as well as in women without pre-eclampsia, and they seem to be narrowed by plaques of cholesterol and blood clots in much the same way as the coronary and leg arteries are in 'ordinary' high BP. This reduces placental blood supply, which somehow induces raised BP throughout the body, with reduced blood flow through the liver and kidneys (untreated, this can lead to kidney failure). The way the blood clots may also be affected and, again, if untreated, blood clotting could be prevented altogether, leading to severe bleeding before, during or immediately after the birth.

All these changes sound frightening but they are rare in modern practice, with regular antenatal supervision and prompt action at the first signs of pre-eclampsia.

I have just learnt that I am pregnant for the first time. How likely is it that I will get pre-eclampsia?

In Western countries about 5% of women expecting their first babies will get pre-eclampsia. In most women it will be in a mild form, but about 1 woman in 250 may get a more severe type of pre-eclampsia.

In some studies as many as a quarter of all women have been found to have some rise in BP during their first pregnancy, instead of the expected fall. However, as we have seen in other parts of this book (especially Chapter 3), the accuracy and reliability of BP readings can be affected by many different things, so these rises may be because of anxiety or the number of different people taking the BP measurements.

My mother and my sister both had pre-eclampsia in their first pregnancies. I've heard that it runs in families, so what are my chances of having it?

We do know that, as with pre-existing high BP, there is an inherited tendency for pre-eclampsia to run in families, which is why midwives and doctors ask you about BP in your relatives, particularly in your mother or sisters. Estimates vary between a 2-fold and 4-fold increase in your risk of pre-eclampsia with any existing family history. The highest risk is where both a mother and a sister had pre-eclampsia leading to a 10-fold increase in risk. Many of these studies are old, reflecting care when women were having babies in the 1930s and 1940s, and their daughters were having their babies in the 1960s and 1970s. Much has changed in the last 20–30 years, so we would expect the chances of developing pre-eclampsia or eclampsia to be fewer today with our improved antenatal care and earlier inductions when pre-eclampsia does occur.

It would be sensible for you to tell your obstetrician and the other people caring for you during your pregnancy about this family history of pre-eclampsia. The more they know about your medical history and background, the better they can look after you.

If I do develop pre-eclampsia, will it harm my baby?

The main risks to your baby relate to poor growth and prematurity. Babies born at a lower weight than expected for the stage of pregnancy may take a while to establish a good feeding pattern and steady weight gain. This may mean additional 'top-up' feeds as well as breastfeeding and occasionally the baby may need to be fed with a small tube passed into its stomach if he or she has difficulty sucking.

Pre-eclampsia may cause premature birth, usually with a birthweight under 2.5 kg (5 lbs 8 oz), or your baby may need to be induced early to protect you, the mother. Either way, depending on the degree of prematurity, this does slightly increase the risk of harm to your baby. Babies who are very immature may need special care in a neonatal intensive care unit. In the very rare cases of severe pre-eclampsia early in pregnancy, there may be a risk of the baby dying or survival with disability.

In my last pregnancy one doctor said I had PIH, another said I had PRH, and the midwife said I had PET. What was going on?

At one time eclampsia and pre-eclampsia were together called toxaemia of pregnancy. There was no attempt to separate several different conditions affecting pregnant women, some of which were caused by problems unrelated to high BP. In recent years doctors have tried to make things clearer (or at least more specific) by trying out different names for high BP in pregnancy. Toxaemia is a term rarely heard today, but pre-eclamptic toxaemia (PET) is still used. Pregnancy-induced hypertension (PIH), pregnancy-related hypertension (PRH), pregnancy-associated hypertension (PAH), hypertension–oedema–proteinurea syndrome (HOP), hypertensive disease of pregnancy (HDP), gestational hypertension and gestosis are names that are all used to describe BP that is raised during the latter part of pregnancy and which gets better after the baby is born.

This is all very confusing to the mother! If we must use abbreviations, the most sensible would seem to be PE (for pre-eclampsia), because eclampsia is real, and is what we are trying to prevent. However, this can be confused with pulmonary embolus (a clot in the lung and also a rare complication in pregnancy). If there is no protein in the urine, then you may well find the abbreviation PIH being used, and many doctors and midwives use PET (pre-eclamptic toxaemia) when there is protein in the urine (there are questions about protein in urine later in this section).

Diagnosing and treating pre-eclampsia

Does a doctor deciding that you have pre-eclampsia depend only on high BP measurements or will I have to undergo other tests as well?

Your BP readings are important but yes, they do take other evidence into account. Pre-eclampsia will be suspected if your BP is 140/90 mmHg or more and is known to have been less than this before your pregnancy began, and/or if there is protein in your urine, and/or if you have some swelling of your whole body from increased fluid (oedema). Although most pregnant women will have some mild oedema (usually affecting their ankles and legs), protein in your urine and more severe oedema indicate that raised BP has caused some kidney damage. These are the earliest changes in the sequence of events that may, untreated, end with eclampsia. Occasionally pre-eclampsia is suspected for the first time because of poor growth of the baby when the midwife or doctor examines your abdomen. Babies in this circumstance are usually very quiet with the mother reporting a marked fall-off in the fetal movements.

You are considered to have mild pre-eclampsia if your diastolic pressure is between 90 and 99 mmHg, moderate if it is in the range 100–109 mmHg, and severe if it is 110 mmHg or more. If you have significant amounts of protein in your urine (most accurately measured on a 24-hour collection of urine), then pre-eclampsia is considered to be severe whatever the level of your BP.

Blood tests may help in determining whether pre-eclampsia has led to disturbance in your liver and kidneys or alteration in your ability to form clots.

Protein was found in my urine at my last visit. Does protein in the urine always mean that a woman has pre-eclampsia?

No. A bladder or kidney infection can also cause protein to appear in your urine, so the urine sample you provide should also be checked for infection. The urine tested needs to be a 'clean catch' or 'midstream' specimen, otherwise the germs that normally live in the vagina may be washed into the collecting tube and cause the sensitive urine testing strips (dipsticks) to give a false positive result. You provide a midstream (MSU) specimen by passing a little urine first before you collect your sample in the container provided.

Sometimes you may be asked to collect all the urine you pass in 24 hours, to measure the total protein lost in your urine throughout the day. This should be less than 300 mg in 24 hours. Some people lose protein from their kidneys from time to time, without this signifying any damage.

Why does pre-eclampsia cause protein to collect in the urine?

Urine normally contains only water with a large variety of rather simple waste products (mainly urea and salt) dissolved in it. Proteins (which are large and complex chemical molecules) are normally filtered out and retained by your kidneys, and so do not appear in your urine. When BP rises for the first time in pregnancy, it rises much faster than 'ordinary' high BP in people who are not pregnant. Even though the actual level of raised BP may not be very high, because it has happened quickly, your kidneys have had less time to adapt to the new higher level and so are more easily damaged. The effect of even minor damage is that your kidneys begin to leak protein into your urine.

The amount of protein in your urine is roughly proportional to the severity of the damage to your kidneys. Your kidneys will recover to the pre-pregnancy state following pregnancy; however, occasionally, women are identified for the first time in pregnancy with pre-existing kidney damage. This will only become apparent if the kidneys have not returned to normal by 6 weeks following delivery.

If I already had high BP before my pregnancy, how can doctors recognize if I develop pre-eclampsia?

Blood pressure normally falls during pregnancy (see the answers to the section on *High BP in pregnancy*) even in a woman who already high BP before she became pregnant (like you). Whatever your starting point, a rise above your pre-pregnancy BP level would be a cause for concern, and would alert your doctor or midwife to the possibility of pre-eclampsia.

For those women for whom good pre-pregnancy BP measurements are not available, then BP measurements taken later in pregnancy can be compared with the readings taken early in pregnancy. Some research suggests that a diastolic pressure rising by more than 15 mmHg or a systolic pressure rising by more than 30 mmHg indicate a cause for concern. Urine tests, blood tests and presence of oedema provide valuable additional information in these circumstances.

My legs became very swollen the last time I was pregnant, so my GP was a bit concerned about pre-eclampsia, but stopped worrying when my BP and urine tests turned out to be OK. Please can you explain what was happening?

In severe pre-eclampsia, so much protein may be lost in the urine that the level of protein in blood falls. The blood cannot then retain all the water it contains; some leaks through the walls of the capillaries (the smallest blood vessels) to other parts of your body, making them swell. Because water tends to fall to the lowest point, this swelling first becomes obvious in your legs.

However, swollen legs are extremely common in pregnancy, and usually have nothing to do with pre-eclampsia. Anything that obstructs the flow of blood up your leg veins can cause raised BP in your veins (not your arteries, and arterial BP is what we are concerned with in pre-eclampsia). Fluid can then leak out of the veins into the skin, causing the same signs of oedema. The most obvious cause of such obstruction is the pregnant uterus (womb), and in late pregnancy some degree of oedema is almost inevitable in almost every pregnant woman. It can happen earlier in pregnancy in women who are overweight, or wear tight clothing, or stand for hours on end.

All these common causes of swollen legs can be distinguished from pre-eclampsia because they are not accompanied by protein in the urine.

Finally, don't forget that if only one leg swells, or one leg swells more than the other, the cause may be a deep vein blocked by a clot, a common and important complication of late pregnancy, which may need urgent treatment. See your doctor or midwife if you think this is happening.

If I do develop pre-eclampsia, is there a way for my doctors to treat it or even cure it?

There is no cure for pre-eclampsia other than delivery. Your obstetrician will need to consider the risks to you and your baby in determining the best timing and method of delivery. In late pregnancy it can be treated by starting labour early (induction) or by a planned or emergency caesarean section (an operation to deliver the baby through the abdomen) before labour starts.

Although severe, rapidly progressing pre-eclampsia can occasionally begin at 24–26 weeks into the pregnancy, but this is very uncommon. Most women who get it develop a mild form of the disease at 34–36 weeks with small amounts of protein in the urine, and diastolic BP (the second of the two BP figures) in the 90–100 mmHg range. They usually do well if labour is induced a little early and deliver good sized babies, who can stay with their mothers on the ward. Babies who are very immature may need special care in a neonatal intensive care unit. Depending on how far you are on in your pregnancy, or whether this is your first or a later pregnancy, labour may be induced either by breaking your waters (called artificial rupture of membranes, or ARM) or by using prostaglandin (PG) pessaries or gel inserted into the vagina. Synthetic oxytocin (Syntocinon) may be used to make the uterus contract if labour does not start after the ARM or PG pessary. This has to be given by a drip into one of your veins. Sometimes this may be given immediately the ARM has been done.

If your obstetrician decides that your pre-eclampsia needs drug treatment, then the most likely BP-lowering drugs to be used are either methyldopa, beta-blockers or a calcium-channel blocker (nifedipine). If these drugs are ineffective, then most obstetricians would use hydralazine (a vasodilator drug) or labetalol (a beta-blocker by infusion – injection into a vein). You will find more information about all these drugs in Appendix 1.

We used to be told that rest in bed was the most important treatment for pre-eclampsia, but obstetricians and midwives today don't seem so concerned about this. Can you explain this?

Research studies have compared pregnant women with pre-eclampsia treated by traditional bed rest in hospital with similar women who simply took things easy at home – they have shown no difference at all in how well women (and their babies) got on. Physical and mental rest are important, but many women get more rest if they are allowed up and about in their own homes than if they are compelled to lie in a hospital bed. However, women with pre-eclampsia who are being treated at home do need careful supervision, and should have their BP measured and their urine tested for protein at least once a day, and should be admitted to hospital immediately if they get abdominal pains or headaches.

Pre-eclampsia and future pregnancy

I had pre-eclampsia in my first pregnancy. Am I likely to get it again?

About 1 woman in 50 with mild pre-eclampsia in a first pregnancy and about 1 in 10 of those who had it severely go on to get severe pre-eclampsia in their second pregnancies. About one-third of all women who had pre-eclampsia in their first pregnancies (regardless of whether it was mild or severe) get mild pre-eclampsia in their second. Or, looking at it the other way, two-thirds of those with severe and nearly three-quarters of those with mild pre-eclampsia have no problems with raised BP in their second pregnancies.

I had eclampsia in my first pregnancy and was very ill. I would like to have another baby but I'm scared that it will happen again. What are the chances that I will get eclampsia next time?

Eclampsia is rare. Of the 10 women who had it in the largest research study so far reported, none had eclampsia in their second pregnancy, eight had normal BP and two had mild pre-eclampsia. If you developed kidney failure because of your eclampsia, then it would be worth asking your doctor to check your kidney function – this will involve doing a 24-hour urine collection test and having an ultrasound scan to check the size of your kidneys. There are also blood tests that check for a clotting disorder or disturbance in special antibodies (antiphospholipid antibody syndrome) that can influence your risk of recurrence of severe pre-eclampsia. If these tests are normal, your risk of getting eclampsia or severe pre-eclampsia are small. You will be advised to see a specialist obstetrician early in a future pregnancy and you may wish to ask for a pre-pregnancy visit to discuss the risks before embarking on a further pregnancy.

I've heard that taking aspirin can prevent pre-eclampsia. I had pre-eclampsia in my first pregnancy, so should I start taking aspirin now that I'm pregnant again?

No, for two reasons. The first (and more obvious) is that self-medication can be dangerous. The second is that a number of clinical trials addressing this question have shown conflicting results. A large review of all of the studies testing the value of aspirin in preventing pre-eclampsia has suggested that the risk of developing pre-eclampsia is reduced by 15% as is the risk of death of a baby (this is a much smaller benefit than was initially anticipated). These potential benefits may be important, but aspirin was only started at around 12 weeks of pregnancy in these studies and the safety of aspirin at earlier stages of pregnancy has not been demonstrated. It is important, therefore, that you wait until the stage of your pregnancy is confirmed and that you take aspirin only under medical supervision.

New information becomes available all the time and you may want to discuss it further with your doctor. There are newer studies suggesting that additional supplements of vitamin C and E may reduce the risk of pre-eclampsia, but again there are concerns about fetal safety as the doses used were quite high. Further evaluation is required and you should not take any medication in pregnancy, even over-the-counter drugs (from a pharmacy or supermarket), without discussing it first with a well informed GP or obstetrician.

Blood pressure after pregnancy

I was put on BP-lowering drugs in pregnancy for the first time. How long will I need to continue with treatment?

This will vary according to how high your BP was in pregnancy and how much BP-lowering medication you needed. Some women will see a rapid fall in their BP over several days following delivery. This may allow you to stop all drugs before discharge from hospital. In other women it is more gradual and you may require ongoing medication for up to 6 weeks following delivery, although the amount is usually reduced over time as your BP comes down. If you had been started on methyldopa during pregnancy, this will be changed to a different drug immediately after delivery, as it can lead to a lowering of mood and symptoms of depression. Occasionally with pre-eclampsia, you may need to start BP-lowering drugs for the first time following delivery or require further increases in your medication, as some women show signs of deterioration immediately after delivery before they start getting better.

Will I still need to visit my obstetrician for BP checking after I have had my baby?

Your obstetrician and the midwives will monitor your BP while you are still in hospital. They will hand over your care on discharge usually to your GP and community midwife. You will need to have ongoing BP measurements at regular intervals until your BP has returned to normal off all medication. If your BP continues to be high after 6 weeks, you are probably demonstrating a natural tendency to high BP and will receive ongoing care from your GP. Your GP will also take your BP into account when advising you on contraception. If you had very severe pre-eclampsia you may be asked back to the hospital for a postnatal visit at 6 weeks to discuss the events in your pregnancy, to evaluate the risk of problems in future pregnancies and to arrange further tests if you are found to have a kidney disorder or clotting problem.

My doctor thinks I will need to continue BP-lowering drugs after pregnancy. I would like to breastfeed for as long as possible – will this be safe for my baby?

The same issues arise for breastfeeding as were discussed for drug treatment in pregnancy (see the section on *High BP and planning a pregnancy*). Very few drugs have ever been evaluated by trials that included breastfeeding women, and most of the information available is from indirect studies and reporting of bad outcomes (adverse event reporting). In general terms, most drugs pass into breast milk in small amounts (the same is true for passage of drugs across the placenta to the unborn baby). The safest approach is to take BP-lowering drugs that are considered suitable for pregnancy. The exception is methyldopa, which can be associated with symptoms of depression and is usually discontinued after delivery. If your BP has been well controlled with a beta-blocker or a calcium-channel blocker (usually nifedipine), you can be reassured that this can be continued after pregnancy with a very low risk of any untoward consequences for your breastfed baby. For other drugs you will need to weigh up the benefits of breastfeeding with the risks to your baby of receiving small amounts of the drug in your breast milk. You will be offered expert advice in this situation.

Contraception

I have been on a combined form of the contraceptive pill for several years. Will this increase or decrease my BP?

Combined oral contraceptives (COCs), are the form of the pill that contain two different hormone preparations – oestrogen and progesterone. There is consistent evidence that shows use of COCs increase BP by about 5/3 mmHg on average. In a small proportion (less than 1%) of women taking COCs, much higher BP may be triggered. Unfortunately this response is difficult to predict. It is not possible to tell which women are susceptible to high rises in BP, and these sharp rises can occur many months or years after initial treatment with COCs.

The small rise in BP is seldom recognized in practice, because the COC is mainly used by young women with systolic and diastolic pressures so low, often around 100 mmHg systolic, that even a rise of 10 or 20 mmHg of systolic pressure remains well below levels that will attract attention from most doctors or nurses.

There are many different contraceptive pills available. Are there any differences in terms of their effects on BP?

There is no difference in terms of different formulations of the COC and high BP. The 'pill scare' a few years ago relates to the risk of venous thromboembolism (blood clots in the leg that can travel to the lung) when different progestogen formulations in second- and third-generation COCs were compared. Some studies have shown that newer, third-generation pills, containing the progestogens either desogestrel or gestodene, are associated with a slight increase in the blood clots when compared with older, second-generation pills containing levonorgestrel. These differences in absolute terms are very small, being 15 per 100,000 women per year of use in second-generation COCs compared to about 25 per 100,000 per year of use in third-generation COCs. When the risk of stroke and heart attacks were compared between second-and third-generation pills, no differences could be found.

I have heard that there is a risk of heart attack or stroke with the contraceptive pill. Is this risk increased if I take the combined oral contraceptive?

There is a small increase in risk of heart attack or stroke associated with COC use. It is for this reason that a regular check of your BP – usually every 6 or 12 months – should be made. In women with pre-existing cardiovascular disease, the COC is not recommended because of the overall increase in such disease.

I have been put on the mini-pill. Does this increase BP?

The progestogen-only pill (POP), otherwise known as the mini-pill, is not associated with an increase in BP. The POP is most commonly used in two situations: firstly, in those women who have taken the COC and who have developed high BP; secondly, in women who already have high BP and who do not want to use non-hormonal methods of contraception.

I already have high BP. Will I be allowed to use an oral contraceptive pill?

If your BP has ever been high enough to cause concern, you should not use COCs. Although the COC is not absolutely forbidden, other choices, such as non-hormonal forms of contraception, should be tried, particularly if you have other risk factors for coronary heart disease – smoking, obesity, high cholesterol, or family history of disease.

In women for whom other forms of contraception are not acceptable, changing to a POP with careful monitoring of BP is recommended. It should be remembered that the POP is a less effective contraceptive than the COC. In younger women (aged under 35 years), who are more fertile and in whom the risk of pregnancy-associated heart attack or stroke is greater than

COC-related risk, then the issue of continuing with a COC or changing to a POP is more finely balanced.

I should still like to go on to the pill. How can I minimize my risk of having a stroke or heart attack?

Nobody should consider starting the pill without a BP check. You should also have a clinical history and examination performed, focusing particularly on family history of stroke and heart disease, BP recording and examination of your heart. In women with no personal history of breast and gynaecological conditions, pelvic and breast examination is not necessary. Secondly, you should make sure that your other cardiovascular risk factors are minimized – most often this means stopping smoking. Lastly, most women begin to consider other methods of contraception by about 35 years of age, usually either in the form of the POP or non-hormonal methods of contraception.

How often should BP be checked in women on the contraceptive pill?

Recommended practice is once every 6 months, although many women who have normal readings have a BP check only every 12 months. The best arrangement is to have BP checked each time a repeat prescription is collected.

Menopause and HRT

I am 51 years old and have just discovered that I have high BP. Is the menopause a cause of high BP?

No. Most women have their last menstrual period between 45 and 55 years. Blood pressure rises with age, and many women consult around this time for menopausal symptoms such as flushes and palpitations, so discovery of high BP can coincide with the menopause, but is not caused by the menopause.

My doctor has put me on HRT patches. Does HRT have any effect on BP?

The use of hormone replacement therapy (HRT) is not associated with an increase in BP. The benefits of HRT relate to reducing the symptoms of the menopause, such as hot flushes, palpitations, mood swings and sleep disturbance. HRT is also helpful in reducing the risk of osteoporosis (thinning of bone density) and subsequent fractures, and has been shown to reduce the risk of colon cancer.

These benefits of HRT have to be balanced against the small increase in the risk of venous thromboembolism, breast cancer and endometrial (womb) cancer in HRT users.

Cardiovascular disease, most particularly coronary artery disease, was initially thought to be reduced by the use of HRT. Unfortunately, recent clinical trials have not confirmed these benefits and suggest that HRT increases the risk of such disease in women who have previously suffered coronary artery disease. The association with coronary heart disease and HRT relates primarily to 'opposed' HRT (containing both oestrogen and progestogen components). 'Unopposed' (oestrogen-only preparation) has not been shown to be harmful or protective in terms of risk of coronary artery disease.

If I already have high BP, is this a reason not to take HRT?

HRT can be used by women with high BP. The main issue is to make sure that BP levels are controlled by means of BP-lowering medication. Because of the potentially harmful effects of HRT on coronary heart disease, you should have your BP checked two to three times in the first 6 months and then at regular 6-monthly intervals.

8
Living with high BP

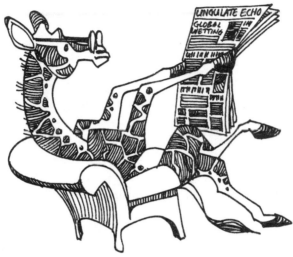

Having high BP can influence many different aspects of your life. In this chapter we deal with the various issues that arise from having high BP affecting different parts of your life, including work, recreation, travel and sex life, and getting personal insurance and a mortgage.

Work

Are there any kinds of work that people with high BP are not allowed to do?

Providing high BP is well controlled by medication, the only kinds of work you cannot do are those excluded by employing authorities, for example flying a plane, scuba or aqualung diving, or other work under raised atmospheric pressure (as in diving bells). These jobs are dangerous for anyone with treated high BP, because all BP-lowering drugs impair the usual responses to the extreme conditions of atmospheric pressure or gravitational force normally experienced in these activities. Anyone with an untreated BP at or over about 140/90 mmHg will be excluded from such employment.

Driving trains or lorries, or operating machinery, might also be barred if you are on BP-lowering drugs that make you drowsy. Discuss this with your GP so that drugs with this side effect can be avoided.

What kinds of work might be bad or dangerous for people making their BP rise? I work in the chemicals industry. Could my high BP have been caused by my work?

This question is difficult to answer, because we still know relatively little about what the environmental causes of high BP are. Some research suggests that sustained industrial noise, at levels that make it necessary for workers to shout in order to be heard over a distance of under a metre (1 or 2 feet), may cause a sustained rise in BP. There is no convincing evidence of any effect from shift work.

Several metals, their soluble salts, or their welding fumes can cause high BP either directly, or by damaging the kidneys. These chemicals include cadmium and lead. The many workers who handle unknown chemicals of all kinds need to be aware of the possibility that these may cause many different sorts of damage, usually to the liver and/or kidney, and this in turn may be expressed as high BP. Carbon disulphide, once used in a now obsolete process for making viscose rayon, was correctly suspected of being a hitherto unknown cause of coronary heart attacks by a vigilant family doctor in North Wales. Other discoveries of this sort may be made in the future; it is sometimes important to keep an open mind.

In studies of Norwegian present and past shipbuilders, both unemployment itself, and fear of impending unemployment, were shown to raise both BP and blood cholesterol. There is good evidence from UK studies of civil servants that lack of job control can have an adverse effect on health but no evidence exists as to whether it influences BP.

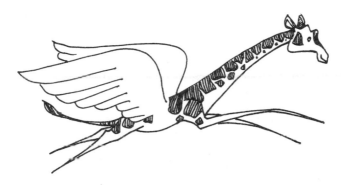

Travel and holidays

Does flying in a pressurized aircraft have any effect on BP?

No, but middle-aged and elderly people with problems of overweight or heart failure should make sure that they have room for their legs without pressure from luggage, that they do frequent static leg exercises by alternately tightening and relaxing their calf muscles every half hour, and get up and walk and stretch regularly on long journeys. Drink plenty of water and avoid alcohol on long-haul flights. There are high risks of developing deep vein thrombosis (blood clots in the veins) in the legs if this advice is not followed.

I am going to Peru soon. Does high altitude have any effect on high BP?

People living long enough at very high altitude to become fully acclimatized develop thicker blood because they need more red blood cells to carry the smaller available load of oxygen. As blood viscosity increases, so does BP and stroke risk. People whose high BP has not yet been fully controlled by medication might be wise to postpone travel to such areas until their BP has been brought down to normal.

Is it difficult to get the same BP medication abroad if I run out?

All the commonly prescribed BP-lowering drugs are available in other economically developed countries, but often at very high prices. Brand names are often entirely different, so you should make sure that you know the generic names of your medication before you go.

Unless you are going away for more than 3 months or so, your family doctor will prescribe enough of your medication to cover the whole period of your absence. If you have to take more than 100 of any tablets for your personal use, it is wise to ask your doctor to write a note confirming what has been prescribed, how much, and that this is necessary for your personal care. Customs officials can be very difficult about bringing large quantities of drugs into countries.

If I need to see a doctor while I am abroad, what should I do?

If you are getting good regular supervision from your own family doctor in the UK, you should avoid interrupting this by seeking other advice, unless this is absolutely necessary. European customs on management of high BP, particularly in France, all the Mediterranean countries, and Germany, differ from the UK and may be confusing. Customs in Holland, Scandinavia and North America resemble our own, although US doctors tend to prescribe branded and newer drugs.

Make sure before you go that you know exactly what medication you are taking, generic names as well as brand names, and roughly what your BP was before you started treatment. It may help to have this written down.

Think carefully before adding any new medication. South and Central European countries have strong traditions of prescribing lots of drugs for everything, which you should avoid. Local doctors occasionally imagine that no tourist can be satisfied with a visit that does not end with a new prescription. Just ask what exactly it is for, and if in doubt, don't collect it. You are more likely to suffer from overtreatment than undertreatment. Lastly, be careful if you take over-the-counter medications for colds or 'flu. Many of these drugs contain ephedrine and caffeine, which raise your BP. It is usually better to take a supply of paracetamol tablets with you.

What should I do about medication if I get diarrhoea or vomiting while travelling?

Travellers' diarrhoea and/or vomiting is rarely severe, and usually self-limiting, getting better after 3 or 4 days without antibiotics or any treatment other than increased fluid intake. Whatever the cause, you should continue your medication unless you have to be admitted to hospital for intravenous fluid replacement, which is extremely unlikely.

Infection with protozoa ('giardiasis') is common in Eastern Europe and the Middle East, and often causes more prolonged diarrhoea and nausea, sometimes dragging on for months unless it is actively treated with the antibiotic metronidazole. This interacts in the blood with alcohol to produce severe headache, but it does not interact harmfully with any of the drugs used to treat high BP.

Diarrhoea is caused by rapid movement in the stomach (gut). Gut movement can be slowed by drugs such as co-phenotrope (Lomotil) and loperamide (Imodium). Either of these drugs is safe to use with BP-lowering drugs.

The main risk from diarrhoea and vomiting is dehydration and depletion of sodium and potassium. Rational treatment mainly depends on correcting these losses by drinking water (drink half a litre – about a pint – after each passage of diarrhoea or vomit). Glucose helps a sick gut to absorb the extra water. You can do this yourself by drinking orange juice or Coca-Cola (for glucose and potassium), adding 1 level teaspoon of table salt to each litre (just under 2 pints); or you can get Oral Rehydration Salts (Dioralyte) from a chemist and dissolve these in water strictly according to the instructions. Make sure that the water you are drinking is pure.

For people on an ACE inhibitor, the normal kidney mechanisms for correcting sudden fluid and salt loss cannot operate. They therefore have much higher risks of collapse, with dehydration and salt loss. For people on ACE inhibitors, rehydration and correction of salt levels must be taken more seriously and medical advice sought.

Sports

I have always done a lot of sports. Now that I have been diagnosed with high BP, are there any sports that are particularly good or bad for me?

Scuba diving may be dangerous for anyone either with uncontrolled high BP, or on BP-lowering drugs. They will have to be satisfied with snorkelling, diving not more than 2 or 3 metres (6–10 feet).

Squash and other similar extremely active and exhausting competitive sports are unwise, and so are all kinds of static exercise such as weight-lifting, press-ups and body-building.

Apart from these, there is virtually no sport that people with treated and controlled high BP cannot do, providing they get themselves sensibly into training, and do not rush into very demanding activities for the first time in middle-age. As discussed in Chapter 4, people who maintain regular exercise tend to have lower BPs. Swimming is probably the best form of exercise, as it remains possible even for older people with joint and back pain. Cycling is a good alternative for people without back pain.

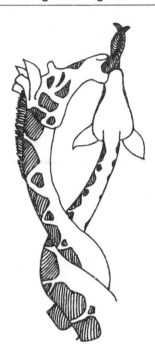

Sex

I am worried that I won't be able to make love to my partner as often as usual. Does high BP affect sexual appetite or performance?

Roughly 5% of middle-aged men, and an unknown proportion of women, have problems of diminished desire and/or performance. There is no evidence whatever that high BP itself affects either of these, but, in any large group of men with high BP, this figure for failure of erection is likely to be nearer 10% or more. This is not because of high BP itself, but because of other factors, such as:

- health changes commonly associated with erection failure, for example diabetes;

- causes of high BP, such as obstruction, for example, of the aorta or of arteries in the pelvis;

- blood-pressure lowering medication, most commonly high dosage of diuretics;

- worry and loss of confidence associated with the diagnosis of high BP.

Sex starts in the mind. If the mind is disturbed or preoccupied with other worries, such as 'Will I (or my partner) have a brain haemorrhage from high BP while we make love?', the sequence of first emotional changes then physical changes, which must occur before successful lovemaking can take place, may not even begin; or, having begun, may at any point be interrupted. Depending on where this interruption occurs, the consequences may be:

- loss of desire or failure to obtain an erection;

- having obtained it, failure to maintain it until both partners achieve orgasm; or

- premature ejaculation.

Although all these failures refer to men, in whom they are more obvious, there is no reason to doubt that they happen also in women, for whom erection of the clitoris is just as necessary as penile erection in men.

Men who usually have good erections when they wake in the morning can be sure that there is unlikely to be a physical problem. Whatever problems they have are probably connected in some way with their own mind, or the interaction between minds necessary for a successful relationship. Problems of this sort can often be solved simply by discussing them frankly with your partner, a simple step many find very difficult to take. If problems can't be sorted out in this way, you should look for help from an experienced and sympathetic counsellor. Local Family Planning clinics and marriage counselling units can usually organize this for you.

Men who rarely or never have good morning erections nearly always have an underlying physical cause, because of problems either with their blood supply or nervous control of the penis. Both these impairments are very common in people with diabetes, often at an early stage in the disease. As diabetes is much commoner in people with high BP than it is in the general population, failure of erection is also commoner among people with high BP.

Erectile failure from a physical cause ('organic impotence') can be treated in several ways. Drug treatment with sildenafil (Viagra) or one of the newer ones (tadalafil [Cialis], vardenafil [Levitra]) enables many men to achieve a satisfactory erection. Viagra should be taken about an hour prior to sexual activity. Adjustment of the dosage may be necessary and you should **not** take it if you are already taking certain antianginal medication (nitrates). If in doubt, consult your GP.

In men in whom Viagra doesn't work, there are alprostadil injections. This drug is injected into the skin at the base of the penis with a very fine needle. This will last for 10–20 minutes, and can be repeated. This sounds awful, but usually works very well, particularly if the main problem is impaired nervous control rather than impaired blood supply, as it usually is in diabetics.

Another choice is the vacuum therapy device (VTD), consisting of a vacuum chamber with a constriction ring, and a hand- or battery-operated pump. It creates a negative pressure around your penis, increasing the blood flow, thus inducing an erection. The constriction ring maintains it.

Finally, you can consider having a surgical operation to implant either a fixed or variable internal splint into the penis, so that you can make an erection. This also generally works very well. The latter two options require referral to a specialist clinic.

Erectile failure caused by BP-lowering medication is relatively common (see Chapter 5), mainly from diuretics (often in excessive doses), beta-blockers and methyldopa, but occasionally with all such drugs. Impotence from this cause is always reversible; it stops soon after stopping the drug. If it doesn't, the drug is not the cause.

Will having sex raise my BP?

Yes, but transiently. As in any other vigorous physical activity, BP rises moderately in anticipation, and steeply during performance. It falls quickly afterwards, and there is some evidence that regular sexual activity may reduce rather than increase average BP at other times.

I already have a high BP. Can sexual activity be dangerous for people with high BP?

Activities that cause very high peaks in BP, such as weight-lifting, push-ups, or pushing a car out of a ditch, are dangerous for people known to have uncontrolled high BP, and unwise even if high BP has been controlled by medication. The risks are of acute coronary insufficiency leading to interruption of normal heart rhythm, and bleeding from a brain artery leading to stroke.

Even if sexual activity were to raise BP to the same extent and for similar lengths of time, this might not carry the same risk. The whole body is in a transiently exalted state during sexual activity, in which perception of pain, for example, virtually disappears; many other changes occur other than raised BP, probably including changes in blood coagulability, which are more likely to prevent than to cause a heart attack or stroke. Coronary thrombosis and heart attack can occur occasionally during intercourse, and stroke is not impossible. However, even these rare events seem to happen far less often during sexual activity than in common and equally physically demanding sports.

I have high BP for which I am taking tablets. I am having problems with getting an erection. What advice can you give me?

There are several aspects to this question. Firstly, taking any medication for high BP does not stop a man using treatments for erectile failure.

The second issue is that some people think that their drug given for high BP has caused the failure. You might have noticed this only when the BP-lowering treatment was started. The real problem, however, lies in the underlying disease, which has narrowed your blood vessels and hence caused your BP to rise, and stop the blood flowing to the penis. **It is very important, if your doctor has put you onto a BP-lowering drug, not to**

stop it if erection failure follows, but to return to your doctor and discuss this issue with him. Your doctor should easily be able to prescribe another drug to control your BP and this could help your problem. It is, however, true that some of the older drugs treating high BP do cause more problems than some of the newer drugs. So your doctor may decide to change your treatment for high BP to see if one drug can control both your BP and erection problems.

Insurance and mortgages

My BP was found to be high at an examination for private insurance. What should I do about this?

The main difference between a BP measurement taken by your own doctor, and by a doctor acting for an insurance company is that your own doctor is more likely to give you the benefit of any doubts. Virtually all insurance companies agree that, if a high BP is found, the examining doctor can let the applicant lie down and rest for about half an hour and then repeat the measurement, using the lower figure if there is one.

Remember that one high measurement does not mean that you have high BP – the single high measurement could have been caused by your rushing to get to your appointment on time, or because you needed to empty your bladder, or for other reasons. If either the examining doctor or your own GP feels that it might indicate a cause for concern, then the answer is for you to have a series of accurate measurements made on separate days to establish whether you really do have a BP high enough to warrant further investigation and treatment (see Chapters 2 and 3 on the diagnosis and measurement of BP).

What if I really do turn out to have high BP, or supposing I knew I had high BP before I applied for insurance? Would it make a difference? Would it affect my ability to get insurance?

Insurance companies are conservative in their habits. Your BP would have to be very high indeed for insurance to be refused outright, but a weighted premium is likely if you are on BP-lowering drugs or if your reading comes close to the BP threshold for considering treatment (such thresholds vary between different insurance companies). Most often insurance companies ask your own GP to provide numerous previous BP readings if they are concerned that you have high BP readings. You can ask your own GP to provide repeated readings if your BP is 'borderline' in terms of reaching the insurance company's threshold.

The British Heart Foundation (address in Appendix 2) can supply you with a list of insurance companies and brokers who understand about high BP and who can help you find suitable policies.

Do I need to mention my high BP on the form for my travel insurance?

Yes, because it is what insurance companies regard as a 'pre-existing condition'. This applies to all forms of insurance, not just travel insurance – it is up to you to inform the insurance company about all pre-existing conditions, whether or not they specifically ask about them. If you do not mention that you have high BP, then your insurance may turn out to be invalid.

I'm 28 and have been turned down for a mortgage because of high BP, but my GP say my BP is not high enough to need treatment. Can you make sense of this?

Mortgage companies, like insurance companies, make their profits by calculating as accurately as possible the probability of an earlier-than-expected death in their customers over the periods of the loans or the associated insurance policies. They make these calculations on the basis of large groups, not individuals – hence their tendency to put people into categories and not consider individual circumstances.

Until quite recently, high BP was generally considered to mainly affect middle-aged or older people (except in women, where it might have been found during routine antenatal care or when starting on the contraceptive pill). In fact most people do have higher BP at younger ages, but their readings fall below the conventional BP threshold or their risk of cardiovascular disease was felt to be too low because of their younger age. Insurance and mortgage companies may not have allowed for this fact in your case and may have based their calculations over a lifetime risk of heart disease or stroke and death.

What can you do about this? First make sure that you really have got high BP, by getting a series of accurate readings. Discuss treatment options, if necessary, with your GP. Finally go back to the mortgage company with your supporting evidence and try again.

Your local surgery

If I've moved to a new area or for any other reason need to change my doctor, how do I go about choosing a new one to treat my high BP? How will the new practice get my medical records?

Your local health authority can give you information about local GPs – who they are, where they qualified and their practice area and so on. It's then up to you to find out more about them; you can always ring up a practice and ask them if they have a doctor who takes a keen interest in high BP. Many practices now issue leaflets that tell you more about the doctors and about the health professionals working there, surgery hours and all the other things you may want to know. If you want to know what other people think about a particular GP or practice, then you will have to ask around – neighbours, people in the post office and local hospitals are all good sources of opinion about local practices, but it is seldom wise to rely on just one person's opinion.

It usually takes about 3 months, but it may take longer, for your new practice to get your records – it depends on the efficiency of your former GP and the health authorities involved. When you move it is probably wise to ask your former doctor to let you have a photocopy of the relevant parts of your medical record or a computer printout of the drugs you are prescribed. You can then hand this directly to your new doctor/practice when you move.

If I am going to be on BP-lowering drugs for a long time, do I still have to pay prescription charges?

Needing BP-lowering drugs regularly does not qualify you for exemption from prescription charges. However, you may be exempt for other reasons – because of your age, because of other conditions (for example, diabetes), because you are pregnant, because you are on income support or a low income. If you are on a low income, you will need to fill in an HE1 form from the Department of Social Security and they will consider your application. If you are not exempt but still paying for a lot of prescriptions, then it may be worth considering prepaying your prescription charges by buying a 'season ticket' for a 4–12 month period. These season tickets will cover all your prescription charges, not just those for your BP-lowering drugs. Before you go ahead and do this, you need to calculate, based on the current prescription charge, whether the price of your season ticket will be cheaper than the cost of the original number of prescriptions in a year that you'll need. If you decide to go ahead and buy one, you will need to fill in the form FP95 available from most doctors' surgeries, pharmacies and post offices.

You may also be interested to know that, at the current cost of NHS prescriptions, some BP-lowering drugs are actually cheaper bought from your chemist on a private prescription, so it may be worth asking about this.

Everyday life

Can I carry heavy shopping?

When you are carrying shopping, most of the hard work is done by your legs, and it's good exercise but tiring. It should not affect your BP. Why not use a wheeled shopping trolley and get your exercise in some other way?

Can I drive safely on BP-lowering drugs?

Some drugs used to lower BP can make you drowsy and this may cause problems for some drivers. Methyldopa and some beta-blockers are known particularly to cause drowsiness. All the drugs that do make people drowsy will do so much more if they're combined with alcohol.

The answer is that, if you feel drowsy on medication, you should discuss with your GP whether you should drive. It is worth mentioning that beta-blockers have been effectively prescribed for people who are nervous and are taking their driving test. They can have a calming effect particularly in people with a tremor.

Are there any support groups or self-help organizations for people with high BP?

Not specifically. There are some organizations such as the Stroke Association and the Blood Pressure Association who provide self-help leaflets and informal support. It is also worth looking at the patient information leaflets produced by the British Hypertension Society. All these organization's addresses are in Appendix 2.

9

Monitoring and follow-up

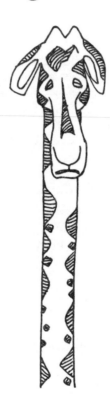

Systematic registration, review and recall is the cornerstone to organized care for people with high BP. Achieving target BP ensures that the benefits of BP-lowering are realized. To achieve this aim you need to be prepared to take part in an organized system of monitoring and care. This chapter describes the key issues concerned with monitoring and follow-up of high BP.

What kind of follow-up should I expect from my general practice? What are the main reasons behind continued follow-up?

It is important that you maintain continuity with your general practitioner so that your BP is properly managed. The aims for follow-up of BP are:

- to make sure that BP is reduced sufficiently to an agreed target level;

- to assess complications of hypertension (target organ damage);

- to continue to assess and treat cardiovascular risk factors, particularly high cholesterol levels;

- to assess possible other illnesses, such as newly diagnosed angina, and consequent tailoring of treatment;

- to continue monitoring any adverse effects from BP-lowering drugs, which may require regular monitoring of your kidney or liver function by means of blood tests.

Your GP may also ask you about how well you are taking your medication and whether you are maintaining your lifestyle changes, such as stopping smoking and losing weight.

If I have side effects with the medication that I am on, will I be able to change?

Your GP should be willing to change your drug treatment when necessary. Your GP will want to discuss with you why you want to change and the choices that are open to you.

Can BP be reduced to too low a level?

BP has a continuous graded and direct relationship with death or illness from a heart attack or stroke. In other words there is no BP level that is too low or unsafe in terms of your overall health.

Several years ago there were concerns that lowering of BP might increase risk of death from other causes. However, when large numbers of people have been followed up over time, the association between low BP and subsequent death was found to be due to the fact that low BP may be caused by other life-threatening coexisting conditions such as cancer. You should not be worried about lowering your BP too much. The problem most people are faced with is not being able to get their BP down to target treatment levels.

I have trouble taking my medicines and frequently miss a dose. Is this a common problem and how can I be helped?

It is well recognized that for symptomless conditions like high BP, people often forget to take their medication. Studies have shown that certain things, such as telephone reminders, more information and better motivation, can help people remember to take their medicines. Adjustment to the dosage of medication that people take can also help – once-daily dosages are associated with better levels of compliance than medications that have to be taken twice or three times daily. Education systems that help people remember and also help people understand reasons why they are taking BP-lowering drugs can also be effective. There are also special containers available from pharmacies to remind you when to take your tablets and to show you if you have forgotten to take your day's dose.

If you are finding it difficult to take your medicines or are forgetting to take them, recognize that this is an important issue that should be discussed with your GP or practice nurse. Often people fail to take their treatment because they suffer side effects. There are alternative treatments available and, if you feel you can't tolerate a particular type of BP-lowering drug, you should discuss the alternatives.

When I am attending my general practice for follow-up care for my high BP what should I expect?

Suggested guidelines for doctors for follow-up and control of high BP follow a graded approach in terms of the frequency of visits until your BP is fully controlled. Initially you should expect to be asked to attend monthly visits for any adjustment of drug treatment until two or more BP readings are below the target treatment level. If you've been recently diagnosed, you may be asked to return once a month until your BP readings are stabilized, you are tolerating your BP-lowering drugs and you have no outstanding worries. For people with very high initial BP readings, or with a history of intolerance to drugs, or with other cardiovascular risk factors or target organ damage, a 3-monthly review interval is recommended. For those people who are well controlled on stable BP medication and with a stable BP reading, 6-monthly visits are usually recommended.

Will I have to undergo any more tests at follow-up other than BP measurements?

Generally speaking two-thirds of people with high BP require two different drugs to adequately control their BP (and reach their treatment target level). It usually takes a minimum of 3 months to make sure that people have stable BP readings, are comfortable taking their BP medication and suffering no side effects.

Blood test monitoring is often recommended to assess kidney function in people taking ACE inhibitors and diuretics. In addition, other conditions such as high cholesterol readings may also be monitored by regular blood tests.

Does it make any difference who's involved in my follow-up care?

There is no strong evidence to suggest that any one professional group is superior to another in terms of managing a long-term follow-up of high BP. Nurses, pharmacists and physician/ pharmacist teams have all been evaluated. All professional groups have produced equivalent outcomes in terms of BP control. Many practices now delegate routine hypertension monitoring to practice nurses and most people find this method of delivering ongoing care entirely satisfactory.

Is there any evidence whether hospital outpatient clinics or general practice is the best place to have my BP monitored and followed up?

There is no firm evidence to suggest either general practice or outpatient clinics are the best place to have your BP followed up and monitored. The main issue concerning BP monitoring is that there is a regular review and recall system ensuring that your BP is monitored consistently over time and that your medication review is regularly checked. This involves you being registered as a person with hypertension who is then contacted regularly to make sure that monitoring and review takes place. Whether this is done in the hospital outpatient department or in a general practice is immaterial. As high BP is such a common condition, most care is delivered in the community through general practice.

I've been told that I've got difficult to control BP. What makes it difficult?

Failure to control BP to target treatment levels is relatively common. It has been estimated that up to 40% of people fail to meet treatment levels (this proportion varies depending on the target level quoted).

There are several factors associated with poorly controlled BP that need to be addressed in a systematic way by the doctor or nurse who is managing your care. These include:

- inaccurate BP measurement

- white coat hypertension

- insufficient treatment

- not sticking to the BP-lowering drugs

- medications that interact with BP-lowering drugs such as non-steroidal anti-inflammatory drugs (NSAIDs), and

- other conditions and diseases that make BP more difficult to control.

If you have poorly controlled BP, your GP should systematically rule out these factors as a cause for it. This often
requires additional blood tests and modification of your anti-
hypertensive medication.

**I have been on some other drugs that the doctor said had
caused an increase in my BP. Which drugs cause this?**

The following substances may be associated with an increase
in BP:

- corticosteroid tablets

- excessive alcohol consumption

- amphetamines, particularly in the form of appetite
  suppressants

- excessive caffeine intake, usually in the form of coffee or
  tea

- non-steroidal anti-inflammatory drugs

- oral contraceptives

- sodium-containing medications, particularly antacids used
  in the treatment of heartburn, and finally

- illicit drugs such as cocaine.

You need to be vigilant to make sure that you are not taking
drugs that antagonize the effects of BP-lowering drugs. This is
another reason why you should attend for regular review so that
your medications and BP can be checked regularly.

**My doctor is referring me to a specialist as he says I have
secondary hypertension. Why?**

As discussed in Chapter 2, secondary hypertension accounts for
less than 1% of the cases of high BP. The main causes relate to

kidney or hormonal disorders. If you have poorly controlled high BP and the common causes of uncontrolled high BP have been ruled out, you will be referred to a hospital specialist so that investigations can rule out or detect rare, secondary causes of hypertension.

10
Research and the future

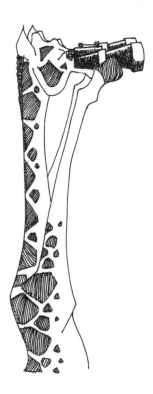

Research into the causes, diagnosis and treatment of high BP continues on a large scale. For the most part research is led by academic institutions or pharmaceutical companies, often in collaboration. This chapter outlines some likely developments over the next few years.

How is treatment of high BP likely to change over the next 10 years or so?

At present a great deal of investment in the different classes of BP-lowering drugs is being made by pharmaceutical companies. There are several thousand people recruited to randomized trials (where people are randomly allocated to receive one or other drug or a placebo, where the tablet contains no active ingredients at all), comparing older and newer BP-lowering drugs with the objective of establishing which, if any, is best. This research is also being run in different people who have different risk factor profiles or other conditions. At present the main four classes of BP-lowering drugs (diuretics, beta-blockers, calcium-channel blockers and ACE inhibitors) are similar in effect. In fact, recent studies from North America have shown that the older BP-lowering drugs are as effective as the newer drugs for most people.

The most likely important change is the reclassification of primary high BP ('essential hypertension') from an apparently single category including all people with high BP of unknown cause, all treated in more or less the same way, into subgroups for which different causes are known, and therefore different treatments are most appropriate.

Are there likely to be any new developments in the genetic aspects of raised BP?

'Genomics' is the term given to the study of functions and inter-actions of the genes in the human genome. There is great interest in linking the function of genes to disease and physiological mechanisms and eventually to effective drug treatments. For instance the renin–angiotensin system and autonomic nervous system (see Chapter 2) are known to play a role in the development of high BP. Scientists are trying to find a genetic link in the hope that drug treatments can be 'tailored' to people with a specific genetic make-up.

I like to surf the net. Is the internet likely to influence research into high BP?

The internet is being increasingly used for dissemination of information about high BP. There are many internet sites that provide information for people with high BP. Appendices 2 and 3 include some relevant websites. It is possible that in the future the patient registers in general practices and hospital clinics may be linked through 'managed clinical networks' on the internet. There are several successful examples in diabetes care. The advantage is that all relevant medications and investigations will be available irrespective of where you may be seen, and communication between health professionals is improved. Ultimately, we will all have an individual electronic health record, that can be accessed through a secure internet connection, allowing access to laboratory investigations and medication records, irrespective of the site of care – in your GPs surgery or in a hospital clinic.

You've spoken a lot about cardiovascular risk throughout the book. How is this likely to change the management of hypertension?

It is likely that prevention of stroke or heart attack will become the starting point and that all risk factors – age, sex, cholesterol, weight, smoking, diet and previous past medical history – will be considered simultaneously. It is also likely that drug treatment will become more 'tailored' to suit the particular risk factor profile of each person.

Glossary

acupuncture A traditional form of treatment in China, acupuncture involves inserting special very fine needles into the skin at particular sites on the body in order to balance the 'life energy' or 'vital force' which the Chinese call *ch'i* or *qi*.

aneurysm A swelling or bubble-like stretching of the wall of an artery.

angina Pain over the front of the chest on exertion (e.g. when walking up hills or stairs), caused by reduced oxygen supply to heart muscle.

anticoagulants Drugs which reduce the tendency of the blood to clot.

aorta The largest artery in the body, leading directly from the heart.

aromatherapy A complementary therapy involving treatment with essential oils, which are aromatic (scented) oils extracted from the roots, flowers or leaves of plants by distillation. Aromatherapy often involves massage, but the oils can also be inhaled or added to baths.

arterial blood pressure The blood pressure in your arteries. Raised arterial blood pressure is what we mean by 'high blood pressure' throughout this book.

artery Blood vessel carrying oxygenated blood away from the heart to the capillary network supplying blood to all parts of the body. Arteries have firm muscular walls and contain blood under relatively high pressure.

arteriole The smallest type of artery, which ends in the capillary network.

atrial fibrillation Rapid uncoordinated muscle activity in the atria (auricles), which are the upper chambers of the heart. It may be treated with drugs to restore a normal heart rhythm and to reduce the heart rate or, in some circumstances, by an operation to insert a pacemaker.

bile A substance produced by the liver which has two main functions.

It helps to break down fats in the gut so that they can be digested, and it also carries away waste products produced by the liver.

blood volume The total amount of blood in your body.

body mass index or **BMI** A way of ranking any group of people with various heights according to how fat they are. It is calculated by dividing your weight in kilograms by the square of your height in metres. A 'normal' BMI value is between 20 and 25.

brachial artery The main artery in the upper arm, used when measuring blood pressure.

brain stem The area lying between the brain and spinal cord which controls many unconscious bodily functions, including heart output, urine output (which affects blood volume), and the diameter of small arteries in different parts of the body (the main determinent of blood pressure).

brand name or **trade name** Most drugs have at least two names: the brand or trade name is the name given to a drug by its manufacturer, and is usually written with a capital first letter. The other name is the generic name, used in all scientific discussion.

caesarean section An operation to deliver a baby through the wall of the abdomen.

calorie Unit in which energy or heat is measured. The energy value of food is measured in calories. If we are to be strictly correct, we should really be talking about the energy value of food being measured in kilocalories (often abbreviated to kcal or written as Calories with a capital first letter), but most people simply use the shorthand term 'calorie' when they mean kilocalories, and that is what has been used in this book.

capillary The smallest type of blood vessel in the body, through which body cells receive oxygen and dispose of their waste products.

capillary network The network of capillaries carries blood from the arterioles (the end of the arterial system) to the venules (the beginning of the vein or venous system).

cardiovascular disease Disease leading to heart attack or stroke. Cardiovascular risk refers to a person's risk of suffering a stroke and/or a heart attack.

cholesterol A fat-like substance which is an essential component of all body cells. Excess cholesterol in the blood may be deposited as plaque on the walls of arteries.

claudication Leg pain from obstruction or hardening of the leg arteries, caused by a shortage of oxygen in leg muscles.

clinical trials or **clinical studies** Scientific research studies into treatments for diseases. They may investigate a completely new treatment, or a new way of giving an existing treatment, or compare a new treatment with older treatments.

clotting factor A substance in the blood which takes part in the chemical processes leading to the formation of blood clots.

coarctation of the aorta A rare condition in which the aorta (the huge artery carrying blood out of the heart) is tightly narrowed a few inches beyond its origin, and then expands to its normal diameter.

complementary therapy A non-medical treatment which may be used in addition to conventional medical treatments. Popular complementary therapies include acupuncture, aromatherapy and homeopathy.

controlled trial A clinical trial in which the group of patients receiving treatment are compared with an untreated or differently treated group, called the 'controls'.

coronary artery The arteries supplying the muscles of the heart with blood.

coronary heart disease or **coronary artery disease** or **coronary disease** Narrowing or blockage of the coronary arteries by plaque. It can lead to angina or a heart attack.

coronary thrombosis Obstruction of a coronary artery by a blood clot. Also called a heart attack.

corticosteroid One of a group of drugs derived from hormones naturally present in the body, which affect the immune system and distribution of sodium and potassium salts. They are used for treating asthma, rheumatoid arthritis and other problems involving the immune system. Although often referred to simply as 'steroids', they should not be confused with the anabolic steroids, which we often hear about being abused by athletes.

cuff A piece of fabric containing an inflatable rubber bladder, which is wrapped around your upper arm when your blood pressure is measured with a sphygmomanometer. Cuffs are available in different sizes to suit everyone from children up to adults with very large upper arms.

depression Feeling sad, hopeless, pessimistic, withdrawn and generally lacking interest in life. Most people feel depressed at some point in their lives, usually in reaction to a specific event such as a bereavement. The most severe forms of depression are often cyclical, occurring at intervals of months or years. These forms of depression seem to arise spontaneously, perhaps because of changes in brain chemistry, and are strongly inherited.

diabetes or **diabetes mellitus** Too high a level of glucose (sugar) in the blood, caused by the body's inability to produce enough of a hormone (chemical messenger) called insulin or resistance of body cells to the effect of insulin.

diastolic pressure The pressure of the blood in the arteries between heart beats. It is the bottom of the two figures in the blood pressure 'fraction' (e.g. someone with a BP of 150/85 mmHg has a diastolic pressure of 85 mmHg).

dietitian A health professional trained in nutrition who can provide advice and information on all aspects of diet and eating behaviour.

double-blind trial A controlled trial in which neither doctors nor patients know which group of patients is receiving the test treatment and which are the controls. This gives more impartial results, as no one's expectations can affect the outcome of the trial.

drug trial A clinical trial where the treatment being investigated is a drug.

eclampsia A rare dangerous condition that occurs in late pregnancy. A woman with eclampsia has fits (seizures) caused by brain damage, caused in turn by very high blood pressure that has developed very fast. Nearly all eclampsia can be prevented by good antenatal care.

embolus (plural emboli) A fragment of material (usually a blood clot) that travels in the bloodstream. Emboli can form in arteries (most commonly the carotid arteries in the neck) and in veins (most commonly deep veins in the legs).

essential hypertension An alternative term for primary high blood pressure.

fetus The baby in the womb.

fibrillation Independent, irregular and uncoordinated movement of the fibres of the heart muscle so that, instead of acting effectively together to squeeze blood through the heart, they tremble or flutter ineffectively, producing irregular, rapid heartbeats.

fibrinogen A substance found in blood involved in the chemical processes that lead to the formation of blood clots.

fulminating An adjective describing any illness or condition that starts suddenly and accelerates rapidly.

generic drug or **generic name** Most drugs have at least two names: the generic name is the scientific name (usually written with a small first letter) and applies to all the versions of that drug, regardless of the manufacturer. The other name is the brand name.

gene A 'unit' of heredity that determines our inherited characteristics, such as eye colour.

genomics The study of the functions and interactions of all the genes in the genome, including their interactions with environmental factors.

genotype An individual person's genetic makeup.

gestosis Another name for pre-eclampsia.

gout A type of arthritis usually affecting the small joints, most commonly but not always in the big toe. It occurs when your body fails to get rid of one of its waste products, a substance called uric acid.

HDL cholesterol or **high density lipoprotein cholesterol** One of the cholesterol-containing substances found in the bloodstream. HDL cholesterol is considered to be 'good' cholesterol because high blood levels predict lower death rates from coronary heart disease. Cholesterol is carried away in this form from the walls of the arteries to be stored in the liver or excreted in bile.

heart attack Death of an area of heart muscle because its blood supply is interrupted, usually because one of the coronary arteries is blocked. The severity of a heart attack (and whether or not it is fatal) depends on the amount of heart muscle affected.

heart failure Inability of the heart to keep up with its work of pumping blood around the body – it fails to pump blood out of the left side of the heart as fast as it comes in on the right side. It does NOT mean that the heart is not beating or is about to stop.

holistic treatment Treatment that aims at treating the whole person (body, mind, feelings, lifestyle etc.) rather than simply responding to and treating individual symptoms.

homeopathy A complementary therapy based on the principle that 'like can be cured with like' (the word homeopathy comes from two

Greek words that mean 'similar' and 'suffering'). The remedies
used (which are completely safe) contain very dilute amounts
of a substance, which in larger quantities would produce similar
symptoms to the illness being treated. Although there is very little
evidence that it has more than a placebo effect and no scientific
explanation as to how it works, it is available through the NHS.
Provision is limited to the small number of doctors who are trained
in its use.

hormone A chemical messenger that circulates in the bloodstream
and helps control the body's functions.

hypertension An alternative term for high blood pressure.

hypertension–oedema–proteinurea syndrome or **HOP** Another
name for pre-eclampsia.

hypertensive disease of pregnancy or **HDP** Another name for
pre-eclampsia.

hypokalaemia Low blood potassium.

impotence Failure of erection of the penis.

induction or **induction of labour** Starting labour and childbirth
early by artificial means, for example by breaking your waters or
by using drugs to make your womb contract.

joule A unit of work or energy in the metric system – the metric
equivalent of calories (one calorie equals about 4.2 joules).

LDL cholesterol or **low density lipoprotein cholesterol** One of
the cholesterol-containing substances found in the bloodstream.
LDL cholesterol is considered to be 'bad' cholesterol because it is
one of the sources of plaque, and because high blood levels predict
high death rates from coronary heart disease.

lipid Fatty substance in the bloodstream including cholesterol and
triglyceride.

malignant hypertension Blood pressure so high that it destroys
arterioles in the retina, brain and kidneys. It is the most serious form
of high blood pressure, a rare medical emergency that occurs either
when very high blood pressure has persisted untreated for many
years, or when blood pressure has risen very fast indeed.

mmHg Abbreviation for millimetres of mercury, the units in which
blood pressure is recorded.

myocardial infarction Another name for a heart attack.

NSAID or **non-steroidal anti-inflammatory drug** A drug commonly used for arthritis, other rheumatic conditions, and generally for pain relief.

oedema Swelling of the body from water accumulating in the tissues. Because water tends to fall to the lowest point, this swelling first becomes obvious in the legs.

ophthalmoscope An instrument, consisting of a special lens on an electric torch, which is used for examining the retina.

osteoporosis Loss of density (thinning) of bone due to ageing. The bones become more brittle and fracture more easily. Women are more vulnerable to osteoporosis after the menopause, because their ovaries stop producing the hormone oestrogen, which helps maintain healthy bones. A calcium-rich diet, plenty of exercise and (where necessary) hormone replacement therapy (HRT) can all help prevent osteoporosis.

palpitation Feeling or hearing your own heart beating fast.

placebo An inert or 'dummy' version of a drug which looks, tastes and smells like the 'real' drug but which contains no active ingredients at all.

placebo effect Most people with an illness or problem tend to feel better after they have consulted a doctor (or another other health professional or professional carer of any sort) and started some plan of treatment (with or without medication). This 'feeling better' is the placebo effect.

placenta The placenta provides the interface between the mother's circulating blood and her unborn baby's circulating blood.

plaque Fatty deposit (consisting mainly of cholesterol and clotted blood) on the walls of arteries that may ultimately weaken or block these vessels.

pre-eclampsia You have pre-eclampsia if in pregnancy your BP is 140/90 mmHg or more and is known to have been less than this before your pregnancy began, if there is protein in your urine and if you have some swelling of your body from increased fluid (oedema). If left untreated, pre-eclampsia can lead to eclampsia. Pre-eclampsia stops when the baby is born.

pre-eclamptic toxaemia or **PET** Another name for pre-eclampsia.

pregnancy-associated hypertension or **PAH** Another name for pre-eclampsia.

pregnancy-induced hypertension or **PIH** Another name for pre-eclampsia.

pregnancy-related hypertension or **PRH** Another name for pre-eclampsia.

primary high blood pressure High blood pressure that is not caused by some other medical condition. It is the most common type of high blood pressure.

pulmonary circulation Blood circulation through your lungs, where it takes up oxygen.

randomized controlled trial A controlled trial in which participants are allocated to receive the active treatment or to be a 'control' on a completely random basis, so that the choice of people for treatment cannot be affected by the researchers running the trial.

retina Usually described as 'the back of the eye', this is the inner surface of the eyeball sensitive to light and colour. All the signals to do with your vision originate in your retina, from where they go to your brain to be organized into a picture of what you are seeing. It has a rich blood supply of very fine arterioles, venules and capillaries. The retina is the only place in the body where the circulation can be seen directly without cutting anything open. This is done by looking through the pupil of the eye with an ophthalmoscope, usually in a dark room or after dilating the pupils with special eyedrops.

secondary high blood pressure High blood pressure for which the cause is known, that is high blood pressure secondary to some other medical condition. Fewer than 1% of people with high blood pressure have secondary high blood pressure.

side effects Almost all drugs affect the body in ways beyond their intended actions. These unwanted 'extra' effects are called side effects. Side effects vary in their severity from person to person, and often disappear when the body becomes used to a particular drug.

slow-release or **sustained-release** or **SR** Tablets or capsules designed to delay absorption of a drug in the gut and so help to supply the drug more evenly through the day.

sphygmomanometer The instrument used for measuring blood pressure.

steroid In this book, an abbreviation for corticosteroid.

stroke Damage caused to part of the brain because its blood supply has been interrupted. A stroke may be caused by a thrombosis in a brain artery, or the artery may have been blocked by an embolus.

Some strokes are caused by haemorrhages (bleeding) within the brain. Strokes may affect movement, sensations, speech, thought and other functions of the brain. Which part or function is affected depends on which part of the brain has been damaged.

subconjunctival haemorrhage A small amount of bleeding in the white of the eye. This may appear after coughing, sneezing or straining when emptying the bowels, and shows up as a bright red area on the white of the eye which then disappears slowly over 6 weeks or so. It is completely harmless.

systemic circulation Blood circulation through the whole of your body other than your lungs.

systolic pressure The pressure at which blood is pushed out of the heart into the arteries when the heart muscle is squeezing. It is the top figure in the blood pressure 'fraction' (e.g. someone with a BP of 150/85 mmHg has a systolic pressure of 150 mmHg).

thrombosis Formation of a blood clot inside a blood vessel.

total blood cholesterol A measure of all the cholesterol in your blood, including HDL, LDL and VLDL cholesterol. An approximate measure of the amount of 'bad' cholesterol in the blood.

toxaemia or **toxaemia of pregnancy** An old name for eclampsia and pre-eclampsia.

trade name Another name for brand name.

transient ischaemic attack or **TIA** Temporary disturbance of vision, giddiness, faintness and confusion lasting for a few seconds and caused by micro-emboli (very small fragments of blood clots) travelling up to the brain, where they break up into minute particles that cause no further problems. They often precede a major stroke and require treatment with aspirin or anticoagulants.

triglyceride The form in which fat is first absorbed from the gut.

uterus The womb.

vein A blood vessel that carries blood back from your body tissues to your heart. Unlike arteries, veins have thin flabby walls.

venous blood pressure The blood pressure in your veins. Although exertion raises your venous blood pressure, this is NOT the type of high blood pressure we are considering in this book, which is high arterial blood pressure.

venule The smallest type of vein, beginning at the ends of the capillary network.

VLDL cholesterol or **very low density lipoprotein cholesterol**
One of the cholesterol-containing substances found in the
bloodstream. VLDL cholesterol is considered to be 'bad' cholesterol
because it is one of the sources of plaque, and because high blood
levels predict high death rates from coronary heart disease.

white coat hypertension This refers to the effect that doctors have
on some people – simply entering a doctor's surgery can make them
so nervous that their blood pressure shoots up. The nickname
comes from the fact that so many doctors (especially those in
hospitals) wear white coats when they are working.

Appendix 1

Drugs used in the treatment of high BP

Group 1: diuretics
(first introduced in 1957)

1A Thiazide and thiazide-like diuretics

1B Potassium-sparing diuretics

1C Diuretics with potassium supplements

1D Loop diuretics

As you can see, diuretics are available in four subgroups. Of these, only those in the first subgroup – thiazide diuretics – are generally useful for treating high BP, and they are the drugs most commonly used today. Use of the others for this purpose is occasionally justified by special circumstances, but in general they should be avoided – if there are special reasons why you need them, you should ask what these are.

Diuretics in general

Although they are very effective BP-lowering drugs, the main purpose of diuretics (and the origin of their name) is to increase urine output. For this reason they are often loosely referred to as 'water tablets'. This can lead to misunderstandings because, although the volume of your urine output will rise when you take them, the frequency with which you need to empty your bladder may or may not rise – so there is a chance that you may think that they are not working when they are actually working well. More importantly, if you are already bothered by the need to make frequent trips to empty your bladder, you may wonder why on earth your doctor wants to make you go even more often.

The main way diuretics reduce BP is probably by increasing output of sodium (salt) through the kidney, although they also widen small arteries and reduce blood volume. They are a little more effective if you also reduce your salt intake.

1A Thiazide and thiazide-like diuretics

When these were first introduced they were mainly intended for treatment of heart failure. They were soon found to be useful for reducing high BP, and have been the mainstay of treatment ever since. They have a few side effects but, because they have been in use for so long and have been so intensively studied, their faults are relatively well understood, and can mostly be avoided by keeping the dose down (they rarely cause side effects unless they are used in unnecessarily high doses). The British Hypertension Society advises that they should be the usual first choice for treatment, and this is endorsed by a large majority of experienced doctors.

The only important differences between the vast number of competing varieties available are the speed with which they work and how long their effects last. If your doctor wants you to have a thiazide diuretic with a slow, steady effect for a once-daily dosage, then you will probably be prescribed chlorthalidone, chlorothiazide or hydrochlorothiazide. Otherwise there is nothing to choose between bendrofluazide and all the rest: all of them will give good control through the day after a morning dose but, if you take them twice daily, you may need to take the second dose in the late afternoon rather than last thing at night, to avoid getting up during the night to go to the toilet.

Thiazides have their full BP-lowering effect at very low doses: if you take more than this, you greatly increase the risk of side effects, without any advantage in reducing your BP. Many doctors, nurses and chemists have still not taken this on board, partly because pharmaceutical companies continue to produce and promote high-dosage tablets. There is ample evidence that it is pointless to take more than 2.5 mg a day of bendrofluazide, 25 mg a day of chlorthalidone (which means half a 50 mg tablet as no 25 mg tablet is currently available), 25 mg a day of hydrochlorothiazide, or 0.25 mg of cyclopenthiazide.

Beneficial side effects

Thiazide diuretics reduce excretion of calcium through the kidney, resulting in two important beneficial side effects. People with a tendency to form stones in the kidney, and women with a tendency to develop osteoporosis (brittle bones) after the menopause, are both less likely to do so if they take thiazides regularly. Multiple fractures from osteoporosis are the main cause of severe curvature of the spine in elderly women, a condition easily prevented but very difficult to treat. The risk is highest in women with a family history of osteoporosis, and who are slightly built with a slender bone structure.

Other side effects

Thiazide diuretics can cause impotence (erection failure), mainly when prescribed in unnecessarily large doses. Reducing the dose to the minimum may help, as side effects are rare at low doses. There is more information about impotence in the section on *Sex* in Chapter 8.

They should not be used in pregnancy, because they cross the placenta and therefore reach the unborn baby, and because they can bring on eclampsia (there is a section on *Pre-eclampsia and eclampsia* in Chapter 7).

There are many possible harmful side effects from thiazide diuretics, but only two of real importance at the low doses recommended. The first is gout; the second is diabetes and glucose intolerance. You will find more information about both of these in Chapter 6.

Their reputation for causing dangerous falls in blood potassium (hypokalaemia) is undeserved, although admittedly at one time this was thought to be a common side effect of thiazide diuretics.

Thiazide diuretics in combination with other drugs

About two-thirds of all people with high BP treated with BP-lowering drugs can only get good BP control by combining two drugs from different groups, usually a thiazide diuretic plus something else. Almost all the other BP-lowering drugs are available as combined preparations, containing a fixed dose of diuretic with a drug from one of the other groups. With the current cost of prescription charges, it can be much less expensive for people who have to pay prescription charges to use these combined preparations. However, because nearly all these fixed combinations contain unnecessarily high doses of thiazides, those who use them are more likely to have side effects than those who take instead the lowest effective dose of thiazide as a separate tablet. (Chapter 8 includes information about prescription charges, exemption from them and prepaid 'season tickets'.)

1B Potassium-sparing diuretics

1C Diuretics with potassium supplements

As was mentioned in the section on thiazide diuretics (Group 1A), low blood potassium was first thought to be a common side effect of taking diuretics for high BP. This concern led to the development and promotion of these two groups of drugs. As their names imply, the potassium-sparing diuretics (group 1B) were intended to prevent excessive potassium loss, while the addition of potassium supplements to diuretics (group 1C) was intended to replace any potassium that had been lost.

We now know that thiazide diuretics rarely lead to low blood potassium in people leading a normal life. For the vast majority of people treated for high BP with thiazide diuretics, low blood potassium is not a significant risk, and none of these drugs should be used routinely for treatment of high BP. One reason for this is that they could cause the level of potassium in the body to become too high (hyperkalaemia). For the large majority of people with high BP who are apparently fairly well and lead a normal life, this danger of high blood potassium now seems much greater than its opposite, low blood potassium. There is therefore a professional consensus that potassium supplements are normally unnecessary, and potassium-sparing diuretics are inappropriate. Unfortunately, they are still promoted for routine treatment of high BP by some drug companies.

1D Loop diuretics

Loop diuretics (of which the most commonly prescribed is probably frusemide) push sodium and water out of the kidneys more powerfully than thiazide diuretics. Unlike thiazide diuretics, they cause a noticeable and often inconvenient increase in the frequency with which you need to empty your bladder, but they are much less effective in lowering BP. They are rightly used for heart failure and in kidney failure, both common complications of long-standing high BP, so many people with high BP are treated with diuretics in this group, but they should not be used routinely to control high BP in otherwise healthy people. Few pharmaceutical companies now promote them for this purpose.

Group 2: Beta-blockers
(first introduced 1966)

After the thiazide diuretics, these have been the next most commonly prescribed group of BP-lowering drugs during the past 15 years or so, although the ACE inhibitors are now catching them up. They work mainly by blocking transmission of nerve messages from the brain stem to the spiral muscle sheath around the small arteries, and by reducing heart output. They reduce BP by slightly less than thiazide diuretics, but by about the same amount as most other BP-lowering drugs. For reasons not yet understood, and unlike other BP-lowering drugs, they seem to have no preventative effect at all against coronary heart disease in people who continue to smoke. There is also some evidence that they work less effectively in people of African descent than in people in other ethnic groups.

Beneficial side effects
A possible beneficial side effect of beta-blockers is a calming effect on nervous people. Beta-blockers have been used successfully to control nervousness in people speaking in public for the first time, in people taking their driving test, and in people undergoing other similar stressful events. They have also been prescribed by psychiatrists to control minor anxiety. In spite of these effects, they are not addictive.

Beta-blockers are also very effective in preventing attacks of angina. This is a common complication of high BP, and there is a section on *Angina* in Chapter 6. For people who have already had a heart attack (coronary thrombosis), beta-blockers have been shown to reduce the risk of sudden death and are routinely recommended in this group of people. Beta-blockers are also effective in reducing the risk of death in people with heart failure. Along with ACE inhibitors, beta-blockers are the preferred drugs of choice in people with heart failure – see Chapter 6.

Other side effects
Unpleasant side effects in some people are tiredness and a generally reduced level of energy, and athletes or people doing heavy manual

work may notice that they become fatigued more quickly. Cold hands and feet are also common with beta-blocker drugs. This is seldom severe and you may be able to avoid it by dressing warmly, and wearing gloves and extra tights or long johns in the winter. The effect may be avoided by combining beta-blockers with another BP-lowering drug that increases blood flow through the limbs, perhaps one of the calcium-channel blockers.

Beta-blockers may cause erection problems and impotence in some men, but the effect soon disappears if the drug is stopped (there is more information about impotence and its treatment in the section on *Sex* in Chapter 8).

Having bad dreams is common in people who take fat-soluble beta-blockers (such as propranolol), which reach the brain. If you have this problem, ask your doctor if you can switch to a water-soluble beta-blocker (such as atenolol), which does not reach the brain.

All beta-blockers slow the heart beat, but this is usually of no consequence. However, people who already have a very slow heart beat (around 60 a minute or less) may get fainting attacks, and so should not use them.

The other serious side effect associated with beta-blockers is bronchoconstriction – narrowing of the air passages of the lung. Because of this effect, use of beta-blockers may be dangerous in people with asthma, but they can be used cautiously in people with chronic obstructive airway disease (chronic bronchitis and emphysema). There is more information about how this is done in Chapter 6.

In summary, beta-blockers are also well established BP-lowering drugs. Clinical trials have shown that they are particularly effective in reducing the risk of stroke.

Different types of beta-blockers may exert different actions on the heart. At present, it is not entirely clear whether these different types of action have important effects in terms of reduction of stroke or heart attacks. Overall, beta-blockers are well assessed and established BP-lowering drugs. They are viewed as 'first-line' drugs suitable for use in most people with high BP.

Group 3: Angiotensin converting enzyme (ACE) inhibitors
(first introduced 1981)

These are relatively new drugs but have been shown in clinical trials to be highly effective – equivalent to older BP-lowering drugs. They are of particular help in certain people – those with diabetes, heart failure, kidney failure and people at high cardiovascular risk. There is now a large choice of different ACE inhibitors available but there does not seem to be much difference between them. As we know more about them, the older ones are probably preferable to their more recent competitors.

These drugs are generally well tolerated, and may be particularly useful for treating the minority of people with high BP who need to start drug treatment under the age of 40. They greatly improve heart function in heart failure (whether or not this has been caused by high BP), and a recent clinical study in the US suggests that they may be particularly effective in elderly people. There is some evidence that people of African descent get a smaller fall in BP from all ACE inhibitors than other ethnic groups.

ACE inhibitors have been shown to be particularly effective in people at high cardiovascular risk. These are people with multiple risk factors that contribute to high overall risk of heart attack or stroke. ACE inhibitors reduce the chance of having such an attack by about a fifth to a quarter. In people at high risk there is a suggestion that the effect of ACE inhibitors may be due to other protective effects aside from lowering of BP. This hypothesis is not fully confirmed, and is the subject of ongoing clinical trials.

ACE inhibitors reduce BP by interfering with the normal mechanism that increases salt excretion by the kidneys when there is too much of it in the body, and conserves salt when there is not enough. This means that the normal mechanisms for correcting sudden fluid and salt loss cannot operate in people taking these drugs, which can cause serious problems if an attack of severe diarrhoea and/or vomiting leads to dehydration. You need to be aware of this if you are on ACE inhibitors, otherwise there could be a risk of you collapsing, with a very low BP and impaired kidney function if you have an attack of diarrhoea and vomiting. You will need to drink extra quantities of water with 1 level teaspoonful of salt and 1 tablespoon of sugar added to each litre (2 pints) of water. You can also make up rehydration solutions based on fruit juice or Coca-cola, or buy sachets of oral rehydration salts from your chemist, and you will find more information about all these in the section on *Travel and holidays* in Chapter 8.

Side effects

The commonest side effect of the ACE inhibitors is a chronic dry cough, which affects about a quarter of the people who take them, women more often than men. In spite of this there is no evidence that they have any worsening effect on asthma.

Captoril (which was the first of these drugs to be introduced) causes a bitter or salty taste in the mouth in about 20% of the people who take it. The taste disappears about 14 days after stopping the drug. Other drugs in this group seem to be free from this side effect.

Otherwise minor side effects are uncommon, but they do present two major risks. Firstly, if ACE inhibitors are started in people who are already taking thiazide diuretics, then their BP may fall so quickly and so far that there is a risk that they may collapse with kidney failure. People already taking thiazides should stop taking them, and leave at least 7 days to pass before starting on ACE inhibitors. Thiazide diuretics can then be added later (if and when necessary). Paradoxically, they are very effective in people with impaired kidney function, but their use usually involves supervision by a specialist. At the early stage, impaired kidney function causes no symptoms; you should always have a blood test first to check your kidney function before you start taking ACE inhibitors.

ACE inhibitors should be avoided in pregnancy because they affect the baby's BP control, may impair the development of the baby's skull, and may reduce the volume of amniotic fluid (the fluid which surrounds the baby in the womb).

Group 4: Calcium-channel blockers
(first introduced 1979)

These drugs impede the transfer of calcium ions across cell membranes, mainly in the heart and arteries (hence the name – they block the calcium channel). However, they have no effect on calcium in the bone, and no effect one way or the other on osteoporosis. Like alpha-blockers, they reduce BP mainly by dilating small arteries. Like beta-blockers, they are also effective in controlling angina, and are often prescribed for this regardless of their effect on BP.

There has been some controversy about the effects of calcium-channel blockers as the different types of drug within this drug class exert different effects on the body. These variable effects include:

- slowing the conduction of the electrical impulse in the heart

- reducing how hard the heart pumps, and

- affecting the smooth muscle tone of the arteries throughout the body.

Some calcium-channel blockers have been shown to be associated with an increase in heart problems and deaths from such, particularly in people with heart failure. These effects have been mostly associated with the shorter acting calcium-channel blocking drugs. For this reason they should not be prescribed to people who suffer from heart failure and probably slow-release forms should be given. Prescribing of BP-lowering drugs to people with different risk factors and other illnesses is discussed in greater detail in Chapter 6.

Side effects

Minor unpleasant side effects are mainly caused by increased blood flow. Flushing and headaches are common with standard short-acting preparations (particularly at high doses), but tend to wear off after a few days in most people. These side effects are much less common with slow-release (SR) preparations, and this is one of the few cases where routine prescription of SR drugs is justified. Ankle swelling occurs in about 10% of people who take calcium-channel blockers, and who are resistant to diuretics.

Calcium-channel blockers reduce the risk of stroke, major cardiovascular events and death from cardiovascular causes but probably less so than drugs in the first three groups. They are particularly effective in elderly people with high BP.

Group 5: Angiotensin II receptor antagonists
(*first introduced 1994*)

These descendants of ACE inhibitors are often called ACE II agents, with the first generation called ACEI. These drugs are related to ACE inhibitors. They have been shown in some studies to be effective in people with enlarged heart muscle (left ventricular hypertrophy). They have been shown to be more effective than beta-blockers in preventing stroke in certain circumstances. Angiotensin receptor antagonists are used primarily as an alternative drug in people who have side effects from ACE inhibitors (usually in the form of a dry cough). Only six have so far reached the market These are losartan (brand name Cozaar), valsartan (Diovan), candesartan (Amias), irbesartan (Aprovel), eprosartan (Teveten) and telmisartan (Micardis).

Group 6: Alpha-adrenoceptor blocking drugs
(first introduced 1976)

Alpha-blocking drugs are used in specific circumstances in people with other illnesses, particularly those people with prostatic symptoms. Alpha-blockers have been shown to be associated with increased illness and deaths in those with a past history of heart failure and they are contraindicated in this group. They reduce BP by dilating (widening) the small arteries.

Beneficial side effects
They improve the flow of urine in men with moderate obstruction from benign enlargement of the prostate. This is common from late middle age onwards, and alpha-blockers can make it possible either to postpone surgery (they improve urine flow about one-third as much as an operation), or sometimes avoid it completely.

Other side effects
The great disadvantage of alpha-blockers is that the first dose often causes fainting unless it is given last thing at night before going to bed. If treatment is interrupted for some reason, this procedure must be repeated. Fainting is rarely a problem after the first dose, except in elderly people (say in their late 70s or older) in whom there is a risk of fainting attacks even after the use of these drugs is well established. Alpha-blockers should not therefore be used for people of this age.

Group 7: Centrally acting antihypertensive drugs
(first introduced 1949)

These drugs – methyldopa, clonidine and minoxidil – act on the brain stem, which lies between the brain and the spinal cord. The brain stem controls many automatic bodily functions, including heart output, urine output (which affects blood volume), and the diameter of small arteries in different parts of the body. Methyldopa (Aldomet) was once the most widely prescribed of all BP-lowering drugs. It remains very popular for treatment of high BP in pregnancy. Clonidine (Catapres) was never widely used in the UK, but is popular in Germany and some other parts of continental Europe.

This class of BP-lowering drug is now reserved for treatment of high BP in pregnancy and they are not generally prescribed in other circumstances.

Side effects

These drugs tend to cause side effects that, although usually only a nuisance, can be intolerable. These side effects occur mainly at high doses and include bad dreams, drowsiness, tiredness, depression, dry mouth and stuffy nose. They can also cause impotence, reversible when the drug is stopped. None should be used for people already prone to severe depression.

Group 8: Vasodilators
(first introduced 1951)

These drugs reduce BP by relaxing the arteries and increasing their diameter. They therefore tend to increase heart rate and heart output unless they are combined with a beta-blocker. They are not generally used in UK practice nowadays. They can cause a strong lowering of BP when combined with either a beta-blocker or thiazide.

Side effects

Hydralazine (Apresoline) may induce an autoimmune disease called lupus erythematosus (LE), particularly in higher doses. This happens more commonly in women than men, and may start months or even years after beginning treatment. LE usually starts as widespread joint pains and swelling, closely resembling rheumatoid arthritis. Unless the possibility of LE is kept in mind, it is easy to imagine that someone has simply had the bad luck to develop another disorder, and to start treating the consequences instead of the cause. Hydralazine-induced LE disappears completely after the drug is stopped, although it may take a long time to go. Hydralazine is also fairly common cause of impotence, reversible when the drug is stopped.

Minoxidil (Loniten) is a last-resort drug for severe high BP, which should be prescribed only by hospital-based specialists. It causes marked hair growth, giving women beards but causing some regrowth in bald men: it is marketed for this purpose as an ointment (which has no effect on BP). Unless combined with a diuretic, it also causes marked water retention and sodium retention and people may develop swollen ankles.

Sodium nitroprusside is given intravenously to control severe or 'malignant' high BP.

Group 9: Ganglion-blocking drugs
(first introduced 1959)

This is a group of drugs that is now used only rarely, and then usually by hospital specialist clinics rather than by GPs. Ganglion blockers work by blocking the nerves that control the spiral muscles around the small arteries, so increasing their diameter.

Side effects

As well as greatly reducing BP, these drugs tend to increase heart rate and may cause flushing. Because the nerve block is applied at the junction (ganglion) between the nerves coming from the brain and the nerves going to the whole circulatory system, their effects are wide-spread rather than concentrated on target arteries and, because the fall in pressure is usually large, they may cause fainting.

Table I Indications, contraindications and side effects
of the major BP-lowering drugs

Drug class	Indications	Contraindications	Common side effects
Thiazide diuretics	Elderly Diabetes (type 2) African–Caribbean ethnic groups	Gout Dyslipidaemia Urinary incontinence	Hypokalaemia Hyponatraemia Sexual dysfunction Gout Glucose intolerance
Beta-blockers	Myocardial infarction Angina Heart failure Migraine	Asthma/COPD Heart block PVD Dyslipidaemia	Fatigue Insomnia Cold extremities Bradycardia
ACE inhibitors	Diabetes Myocardial infarction Angina Heart failure Chronic renal disease*	Pregnancy Renovascular disease PVD†	Cough First dose hypotension Taste disturbance Angio-oedema

Calcium channel
  blockers
	Elderly
	Angina
	Pregnancy
	African Caribbean
	  ethnic groups
		Myocardial infarction‡
		Heart failure‡
			Constipation
			Peripheral oedema
			Flushing
			Headache

Alpha-blockers	Prostatism	Heart failure Urinary incontinence Postural hypotension	Nasal stuffiness Dizziness Postural hypotension
Central agents (methyldopa)	Pregnancy	Postural hypotension	Depression Haemolytic anaemia

Angiotensin
  receptor
  antagonisists
	Intolerance
	  to other drugs
	Heart failure
		Pregnancy
		PVD
			Angio-oedema
			Renovascular disease

Abbreviations: COPD, chronic obstructive pulmonary disease; PVD, peripheral vascular disease.

*ACE inhibitors need to be used with caution in chronic kidney disease as they may precipitate renal failure; people on ACE inhibitors require regular supervision and specialist advice.

† PVD is frequently associated with renovascular disease.

‡ Amlodipine (long-acting dihydropyridine) can be used; other calcium channel blockers are best avoided.

Appendix 2
Useful addresses

Action on Pre-Eclampsia
84–88 Pinner Road
Harrow HA1 4HZ
Helpline: 020 8427 4217
Tel: 020 8863 3271
Fax: 020 8424 0653
Website: www.apec.org.uk
*Offers information leaflets on the
risk of pre-eclampsia. Supports
sufferers and their families and
runs study days for midwives and
health professionals.*

**Aromatherapy Organizations
Council**
PO Box 6522
Desborough
Kettering NN14 2YX
Tel: 0870 774 3477
Fax: 0870 774 3477
Website: www.aocuk.net
*Umbrella body representing
aromatherapy associations. Can
provide details of local therapists,
training and general information.*

Arthritis Care
18 Stephenson Way
London NW1 2HD
Helpline: 020 7380 6555
Tel: 020 7380 6500
Fax: 020 7380 6505
Website: www.arthritiscare.org.uk
*Provides information, counselling,
training and social contact. The
first port of call for anyone with
arthritis, including gout. Many
smaller organizations for
particular types of arthritis; for
details ring helpline or Freephone
0808 800 4050.*

Arthritis Research Campaign
Copeman House
St Marys Court
St Marys Gate
Chesterfield S41 7TD
Helpline: 0870 850 5000
Tel: 01246 558033
Fax: 01246 558007
Website: www.arc.org.uk
*The leading arthritis research
organization in the UK, funding
much research and producing
useful information for patients.*

ASH (Action on Smoking and Health)
102 Clifton Street
London EC2A 4HW
Helpline: 0800 169 0169
Tel: 020 7739 5902
Fax: 020 7613 0531
Website: www.ash.org.uk
National organization with local branches. Campaigns on antismoking policies. Offers free information on website or for sale from H.Q. Catalogue on request.

Association of Qualified Curative Hypnotherapists
PO Box 9989
Birmingham B14 4WA
Tel: 0121 693 1223
Fax: 0121 693 1223
Website: www.aqch.org
Organization representing qualified curative hypno-therapists. Can recommend appropriate courses for training in this field.

BackCare (formerly National Back Pain Association)
16 Elmtree Road
Teddington
Middlesex TW11 8ST
Tel: 020 8977 5474
Fax: 020 8943 5318
Website: www.backcare.org.uk
Offers information and advice about back pain. Has local self-help support groups.

Blood Pressure Association
60 Cranmer Terrace
London SW17 0QS
Tel: 020 8772 4994
Fax: 020 8772 4999
Website: www.bpassoc.org.uk
Offers information and fact sheets about high blood pressure and the various ways it can be treated. An SAE A4 size envelope requested with 2 first class stamps.

British Acupuncture Council
63 Jeddo Road
London W12 9HQ
Tel: 020 8735 0400
Fax: 020 8735 0404
Website: www.acupuncture.org.uk
Professional body offering lists of qualified acupuncture therapists.

British Cardiac Society
9 Fitzroy Square
London W1T 5HW
Tel: 020 7383 3887
Fax: 020 7388 0903
Website: www.bcs.com

British Dietetic Association
5th Floor
Charles House
148–149 Great Charles Street
Birmingham B3 3HT
Tel: 0121 200 8080
Fax: 0121 200 8081
Website: www.bda.uk.com
Professional association supporting dietitians.

British Heart Foundation (BHF)
14 Fitzhardinge Street
London W1H 6DH
Helpline: 08450 708070
Tel: 020 7935 0185
Fax: 020 7486 5820
Website: www.bhf.org.uk
Funds research, promotes education and raises money to buy equipment to treat heart disease. List of publications, posters and videos; send s.a.e. Their helpline, HeartstartUK can arrange training in emergency life-saving techniques for lay people.

British Herbal Medicine Association
1 Wickham Road
Boscombe
Bournemouth BH7 6JX
Tel: 01202 433691
Fax: 01202 417079
Website: www.bhma.info
Offers information, encourages research and promotes high quality standards. Advises members on legalities for importers, vets advertisements and defends the right of the public to choose herbal medicines and be able to obtain them freely.

British Holistic Medical Association
59 Lansdowne Place
Hove BN3 1FL
Tel: 01273 725951
Fax: 01273 725951
Website: www.bhma.org
Promotes awareness of the holistic approach to health among practitioners and the public through publications, self-help tapes, conferences and a network of local groups.

British Homeopathic Association
15 Clerkenwell Close
London EC1R 0AA
Tel: 020 7566 7800
Fax: 020 7566 7815
Website: www.trusthomeopathy.org
Professional body offering lists of qualified homeopathic practitioners.

British Hypertension Society
Website: www.bhsoc.org

British Medical Acupuncture Society
12 Marbury House
Higher Whitley
Warrington WA4 4QW
Tel: 01925 730727
Fax: 01925 730492
Website:
www.medical-acupuncture.co.uk
Professional body offering training to doctors and list of accredited acupuncture practitioners.

British Society of Medical and Dental Hypnosis
28 Dale Park Gardens
Cookridge
Leeds LS16 7PT
Tel: 07000 560309
Fax: 07000 560309
Website: www.bsmdh.com.
Professional body offering hypnosis training to doctors and dentists. Can provide list of accredited local medical and dental hynotherapists.

British Wheel of Yoga
25 Jermyn Street
Sleaford NG34 7RU
Tel: 01529 306851
Fax: 01529 303233
Website: www.bwy.org.uk
Professional body offering lists of qualified yoga therapists. Also provides training courses in yoga.

Chest, Heart and Stroke Association (N. Ireland)
21 Dublin Road
Belfast BT2 7HB
Helpline: 08457 697299
Tel: 02890 320184
Fax: 02890 333487
Website: www.nichsa.com
Funds research and provides information on chest, heart and stroke-related illnesses.

Chest, Heart and Stroke Scotland
65 North Castle Street
Edinburgh EH2 3LT
Tel: 0131 225 6963
Fax: 0131 220 6313
Website: www.chss.org.uk
Funds research and provides information on chest, heart and stroke-related illnesses.

Citizens Advice (National Association – NACAB)
Myddleton House
115–123 Pentonville Road
London N1 9LZ
Tel: 020 7833 2181
Fax: 020 7833 4371
Website: www.citizensadvice.org.uk
HQ of national charity offering a wide variety of practical, financial and legal advice. Network of local branches throughout the UK listed in phone books and in Yellow Pages under Counselling and Advice.

Citizens Advice North Wales
Unit 7
St Asaph Business Park
Richard Davies Road
St Asaph
Denbighshire LL17 0LJ
Tel: 0174 558 6400
Fax: 0174 558 5554
Website: www.adviceguide.org.uk
Offers a wide range of practical, financial and legal advice through local branches, in both English and Welsh languages.

Citizens Advice Scotland
Spectrum House
2 Powderhall Road
Edinburgh EH7 4GB
Tel: 0131 550 1000
Fax: 0131 550 1001
Website: www.cas.org.uk
Provides details of local Citizens Advice branches, which are also available in local telephone directories.

Community Health Council
The address and telephone number of your local CHC will be in the Phone Book
and in Yellow Pages
Website: www.achcew.org.uk
Statutory information service offering advice to users of the National Health Service. Local branches.

Complementary Medical Association
11 Albery Road
St Leonards-on-Sea TN38 0LP
Tel: 01424 438 801
Fax: 0845 129 8435
A not-for-profit medical body offering membership to highly qualified practitioners of complementary medicine. Has database of accredited practitioners around the UK.

Consumers' Association
2 Marylebone Road
London NW1 4DF
Helpline: 0845 307 4000
Tel: 020 7486 5544
Fax: 020 7770 7600
Website: www.which.net
Campaigns on behalf of consumers and produces reports on products including foods.

Coronary Prevention Group (CPG)
London School of Hygiene and Tropical Medicine
2 Taviton Street
London WC1H 0BT
Tel: 020 7927 2125
Fax: 020 7927 2127
Website: www.healthnet.org.uk
First British charity devoted to prevention of coronary heart disease. Produces booklets and fact sheets available on the website or by post. Please send SAE.

Department of Health (DoH)
PO Box 777
London SE1 6XH
Helpline: 0800 555777
Tel: 020 7210 4850
Fax: 01623 724524
Website: www.doh.gov.uk
Textphone: 020 7210 5025
Produces literature about health issues, available via helpline. A more technical site with National Service Frameworks available from internet, e.g. www.doh.gov.uk/nsf/bloodpressure

Diabetes UK
10 Parkway
London NW1 7AA
Helpline: 020 7424 1030
Tel: 020 7424 1000
Fax: 020 7424 1001
Website: www.diabetes.org.uk
Textline 020 7424 1888
*Provides advice and information
on diabetes; has local support
groups.*

Health Development Agency
Holborn Gate
330 High Holborn
London WC1V 7BA
Helpline: 0870 121 4194
Tel: 020 7430 0850
Fax: 020 7061 3390
Website: www.hda-online.org.uk
*Formerly Health Education
Authority; now only deals with
research. Publications on health
matters can be ordered via
helpline.*

**Heart UK (formerly Family
Heart Association)**
7 North Road
Maidenhead SL6 1PE
Tel: 01628 628638
Fax: 01628 628698
Website: www.heartuk.org.uk
*Will help anyone at high risk of
heart attack, but specializes in
inherited conditions causing high
cholesterol (i.e. familial
hypercholesterolaemia)*

**Institute for Complementary
Medicine**
PO Box 194
London SE16 7QZ
Tel: 020 7237 5165
Fax: 020 7237 5175
Website: www.icmedicine.co.uk
*Umbrella group for
complementary medicine
organizations. Offers informed,
safe choice to public, British
register of practitioners and refers
to accredited training courses.
S.a.e. requested for information.*

**International Federation of
Aromatherapists**
182 Chiswick High Road
Chiswick
London W4 1PP
Tel: 020 8742 2605
Fax: 020 8742 2606
Website: www.ifaroma.org
*Professional body offering lists of
qualified aromatherapists.*

**Internatational Society of
Professional Aromatherapists**
82 Ashby Road
Hinckley
Leics. LE10 1SN
Tel: 0145 563 7987
Fax: 0145 589 0956
Website: www.isparoma.org
*Professional body offering lists of
professional aromatherapists.*

Irish Heart Foundation
4 Clyde Road
Ballsbridge
Dublin 4
Tel: 0035316685001
Fax: 0035316685896
Website: www.irishheart.ie
Offers information, publications,
training and support in
prevention of heart disease.
Collaborates with other heart-
related organizations and has
some local support groups.

MIND (National Association for
Mental Health)
Granta House
15–19 Broadway
London E15 4BQ
Helpline: 0845 766 0163
Tel: 020 8519 2122
Fax: 020 8522 1725
Website: www.mind.org.uk
Mental health organization
working for a better life for
everyone experiencing mental
distress. Offers support via local
branches. Publications available
on 020 8221 9666.

National Asthma Campaign
Providence House
Providence Place
London N1 0NT
Helpline: 0845 01 02 03
Tel: 020 7226 2260
Fax: 020 7704 0740
Website: www.asthma.org.uk
Funds research and produces a
range of information about coping
with asthma. Helpline staffed by
team of specialist asthma nurses
who offer good advice on all

aspects of asthma, including
steroid use. Has local support
groups.

National Institute of Medical
Herbalists
56 Longbrook Street
Exeter EX4 6AH
Tel: 01392 426022
Fax: 01392 498963
Website: www.nimh.org.uk
Professional body representing
qualified, practising medical
herbalists. Offers lists of
accredited medical herbalists.
S.A.E. requested.

NHS Direct (formerly Health
Information First)
Helpline: 0845 4647
Tel: 020 8867 1367
Website: www.nhsdirect.nhs.uk
NHS Direct is a 24 hour helpline
offering confidential healthcare
advice, information and referral
service 365 days of the year. A
good first port of call for any
health advice. Textphone for people
with a hearing impairment 0845
606 4647.

NHS Scotland (formerly Health
Education for Scotland)
Woodburn House
Canaan Lane
Edinburgh EH10 4SG
Tel: 0131 536 5500
Fax: 0131 536 5501
Website: www.hebs.scot.nhs.uk
NHS health education board for
Scotland.
Textphone 0131 536 5503

Patients Association
PO Box 935
Harrow HA1 3YJ
Helpline: 0845 608 4455
Tel: 020 8423 9111
Fax: 020 8423 9119
Website:
www.patients-association.com
*Provides advice on patients'
rights. Leaflets and directory of
self-help groups available.*

**Pharmaceutical Association of
GB**
1 Lambeth High Street
London SE1 7JN
Tel: 020 7735 9141
Fax: 020 7735 7629
Website: www.rpsgb.org.uk

Quit
211 Old Street
London EC1V 9NR
Helpline: 0800 002200
Tel: 020 7251 1551
Fax: 020 7251 1661
Website: www.quit.org.uk
*Offers advice to stop smoking in
English and Asian languages; also
to schools, and on pregnancy.
Runs training courses for health
professionals. Can put people in
touch with local support groups.*

**Rare Unspecified Disorders
Support Group**
PO Box 2189
Caterham CR3 5GN
Tel: 01883 330766
Fax: 01883 330766
Website: www.rarechromo.org
*A support group for families with
rare chromosomal disorders.
Produces family-friendly
information and has database of
world-wide matching families.
Confidential discussion forum on
website for members. Database
available to geneticists.*

Relate (Marriage Guidance)
Herbert Gray College
Little Church Street
Rugby CV21 3AP
Helpline: 0845 130 4010
Tel: 01788 573241
Fax: 01788 535007
Website: www.relate.org.uk
*Offers relationship counselling
via local branches. Relate
publications on health, sexual,
self-esteem, depression,
bereavement and remarriage
issues available from bookshops,
libraries or via website.*

Society of Homeopaths
4a Artizan Road
Northampton NN1 4HU
Tel: 01604 621400
Fax: 01604 622622
Website: www.homeopathy-soh.org
*Professional body, offers lists of
accredited homeopathic therapists
and free general information.*

Sport England
16 Upper Woburn Place
London WC1H 0QP
Tel: 020 7273 1500
Fax: 020 7273 1868
Website: www.sportengland.org
*Government agency promoting
sport in England with a wide
variety of activity programmes in
order to foster a healthier lifestyle.*

Stroke Association
Stroke House
240 City Road
London EC1V 2PR
Helpline: 0845 303 3100
Tel: 020 7566 0300
Fax: 020 7490 2686
Website: www.stroke.org.uk
*Funds research and provides
information now specializing in
stroke only. Publications can be
ordered from 01604 623 933.*

**The Royal National Institute for
the Blind**
105 Judd Street
London WC1H 9NE
Helpline: 0845 766 9999
Tel: 020 7388 1266
Fax: 020 7388 2034
Website: www.rnib.org.uk
*Offers a range of information and
advice on lifestyle changes and
employment for people facing loss
of sight. Also offers support and
training in braille. Has mail order
catalogue of useful aids.*

**Vegetarian Society of the
United Kingdom**
Parkdale
Dunham Road
Altrincham
Cheshire WA14 4QG
Tel: 0161 925 2000
Fax: 0161 926 9182
Website: www.vegsoc.org
*Offers information on the
vegetarian way of life, day and
residential training courses at
own Centre. Provides literature for
GCSE projects, advice to school
caterers. Food manufacturers and
restaurants can apply for
vegetarian accreditation.*

Womens Health
52 Featherstone Street
London EC1Y 8RT
Helpline: 0845 125 5254
Tel: 020 7251 6333
Fax: 020 7250 4152
Website:
www.womenshealthlondon.org.uk
*Provides information on
gynaecological and sexual issues
to help women make informed
decisions about their health,
and a range of publications
and quarterly newsletter.
To use reference library, please
telephone first.*

Women's Health Concern (WHC)
PO Box 2126
Marlow SL7 2RY
Helpline: 01628 483612
Tel: 01628 488065
Fax: 01628 474042
Website: womens-health-concern.org
National charity that offers help to women, particularly on questions of hormone health, HRT and gynaecology.

Yoga for Health Foundation
Ickwell Bury
Biggleswade SG18 9EF
Tel: 01767 627271
Fax: 01767 627266
Website:
www.yogaforhealthfoundation.co.uk
Offers teacher training for remedial yoga at their own residential centre for people with health problems.

Appendix 3
Useful publications
and websites

Publications

At the time of writing, most of the publications listed here were available. For current prices, please check with your local bookshop or with the publisher. Your local library may have copies of some of the older books mentioned, and you may well find some of the leaflets available in your GP's surgery, or your local health centre.

Food and cooking

The Everyday Light-Hearted Cookbook, by Anne Lindsay, published by Grub Street/British Heart Foundation (1994)
ISBN 0 948817 78 X

Healthy Eating on a Plate, by Janette Marshall, published by Vermillion (1995)
ISBN 0 09 180857 X

The Light-Hearted Cookbook: recipes for a healthy heart, by Anne Lindsay, published by Grub Street/British Heart Foundation (1999)
ISBN 1 902304 15 2

Which? Way to a Healthier Diet, by Judy Byrne, published by the Consumers' Association/Hodder Headline (1993)
ISBN 0 34 059101 3

The **British Heart Foundation** (address in Appendix 2) publishes a number of free booklets and leaflets on healthy eating – titles include *Cut the Saturated Fat from Your Diet*; *Eating for your Heart*.

The **Health Development Agency** publishes *Enjoy Fruit and Veg* and *Enjoy Healthy Eating*. These leaflets are now available via the Food Standards Agency.

Stopping smoking

Allen Carr's Easy Way to Stop Smoking, by Allen Carr, published by Penguin (1999)
ISBN 0 14 027763 3

How to Stop Smoking and Stay Stopped for Good, by Gillian Riley, published by Vermilion (2003)
ISBN 0 09 188776 3

Kick it! Stop smoking in five days, by Judy Perlmutter, published by Berkley Publishing Group (1998)
ISBN 0 72251 523 5

Stop Smoking for Good with the National Health Association Stop Smoking Programme, by Robert Brynin, published by Hodder & Stoughton General (1995)
ISBN 0 34063 240 2

The **British Heart Foundation** publishes a free leaflet called *Smoking and Your Heart*, which includes advice on how to give up.

The **Health Development Agency** publishes booklets and leaflets on stopping smoking – titles include *Stopping Smoking Made Easier* and *Thinking about Stopping* available via the Department of Health.

Exercise

The **British Heart Foundation** publishes free leaflets on suitable types of exercise such as *Put your Heart into Walking*

The **Health Development Agency** publishes leaflets on exercise such as *Getting Active, Feeling Good* and *Exercise: Why Bother?* These leaflets are now supplied by the British Heart Foundation.

Other relevant topics

Diabetes – the 'at your fingertips' guide, by Professor Peter Sönkson, Dr Charles Fox and Sue Judd, published by Class Publishing (5th edn 2003)
ISBN 1 85959 087 X

Heart Health – the 'at your fingertips' guide, by Dr Graham Jackson, published by Class Publishing (1998; 3rd edn due 2004)
ISBN 1 85959 097 7

The Pill and Other Forms of Hormonal Contraception, by John Guillebaud, published by Oxford University Press (1997)
ISBN 0 19286 188 3

Stop that heart attack! by
Dr Derrick Cutting, published by
Class Publishing (3rd edn 2004)
ISBN 1 85959 096 9

Understanding Stress, by
Professor Greg Wilkinson,
published by Family Doctor
Publications (2000)
ISBN 1 89820 591 4

The **Coronary Prevention
Group's** publication *Stress and
Your Heart* is available either
via their address as listed in
Appendix 2, or can be
downloaded from their website:
http://www.healthnet.org.uk/

The **Department of Health**
publishes *Traveller's Guide to
Health* available at any main post
office.

The **Health Development
Agency** publishes *Cutting Down
Your Drinking; That's the Limit*
and *Women and Drinking*. These
leaflets are now available via the
Department of Health.

Websites

Cardiovascular risk score (based
on individual patient data from
randomised trials):
www.riskscore.org.uk

Individuals' experiences with
illness, including high BP:
dipex.co.uk/EXEC

Joint National Committee on
Prevention, Detection, Evaluation
and Treatment of High Blood
Pressure (US guidelines):
www.nhlbi.nih.gov/guidelines/
hypertension/jncintro.htm

New Zealand cardiovascular risk
charts (based on the Framingham
risk equation):
www.cebm.net/prognosis.asp

Patients facing a treatment
decision:
www.med-decisions.com/cvtool

WHO Guidelines, 1999:
www.who.int/ncd/cvd/ht_guide.html

Useful addresses and websites for important educational materials:

Action on Smoking & Health (ASH)
www.ash.org

Blood Pressure Association
www.bpassoc.org.uk

British Hypertension Society
www.bhsoc.org

National Electronic Library for Health
www.nelh.nhs.uk

Scottish Health on the Web
www.show.scot.nhs.uk

Index

asthma *continued*
BP-lowering drugs and xv
multiple drugs and 86
smoking and 73
atenolol, safety in pregnancy 108
atorvastatin 98
atrial fibrillation 28, 156*g*
BP measurements and 56
herbal products and 33
high BP and 94
atrial sinus 28
autonomic nervous system,
overactive 2, 29

babies
early delivery 122
of pre-eclamptic mothers
117–18, 122
bananas 67
beans 65
bed rest in pre-eclampsia 123
beer-drinker's belly 79
bendrofluazide 167
causing erection failure 100
beta-blockers 170–1, 178
in angina 93
for asthma, high BP and 99
causing erection failure 100,
139
in diabetes and high BP 96
following pregnancy 126
in heart failure 93
for pre-eclampsia 122
in raised lipid profiles 98
response in African-Caribbean
race 101
safety in pregnancy 108
side effects 83, 145, 170–1
stopping treatment 89
bile 156*g*
birth weight and high BP 29

bladder fullness causing raised
BP 50
bleeding into stomach from
aspirin 100–1
blood
cholesterol levels
see cholesterol
clotting
exercise and 74
in pre-eclampsia 116
sex and 140
fats *see* LDL; cholesterol; HDL;
lipids; VLDL
flow 12–13
moving around body 8, 12
supply to placenta 111
transporting materials around
body 8, 110
viscosity 10
at high altitude 133–4
volume 10, 157*g*
kidney role in 97
placental role during
pregnancy 110
blood pressure
effects of COC 127–9
falling during sleep xii–xiii
figures
meaning 10–11
measurement 10–11
in pre-eclampsia 119, 121
in pregnancy 110, 112
ranges in 11
reduction by drugs 84
following pregnancy 125–6
high *see* high blood pressure
low 4, 15
measurement 52
during pregnancy 109–10
lowering to dangerous level
147–8

Have you found **High Blood Pressure – the 'at your fingertips'
guide** practical and useful? If so, you may be interested in other
books from Class Publishing.

Heart Health – the 'at your fingertips' guide
THIRD EDITION   £14.99
Dr Graham Jackson
This practical handbook, written by a
leading cardiologist, answers all your
questions about heart conditions. It tells
you all about you and your heart; how to
keep your heart healthy, or if it has been
affected by heart disease – how to make
it as strong as possible.

> 'Those readers who want to know
> more about the various treatments for
> heart disease will be much
> enlightened.' – *Dr James Le Fanu,
> Daily Telegraph*

Diabetes – the 'at your fingertips' guide
FIFTH EDITION   £14.99
*Professor Peter Sönksen, Dr Charles Fox
and Sue Judd*
This practical handbook makes it easy for
you to learn more about your diabetes –
and the more you know, the easier it is to
manage. This updated fifth edition is an
invaluable reference guide for people
living with diabetes, and offers practical
advice on every aspect of living with the
condition, giving you the knowledge and
reassurance you need to deal confidently
with you diabetes.

> 'I have no hesitation in commending
> this book . . .' – *Sir Steve Redgrave,
> Vice President, Diabetes UK*

Sexual Health for Men – the 'at your fingertips' guide
NEW TITLE   £14.99
Dr Philip Kell and Vanessa Griffiths
This practical handbook answers
hundreds of real questions from men with
erectile dysfunction and their partners. Up
to 50% of the population aged over 60 is
impotent – though they need not be, if
they take appropriate action.

Stop that heart attack!
THIRD EDITION   £14.99
Dr Derrick Cutting
The easy, drug-free and medically
accurate way to cut your risk of having a
heart attack dramatically.

Even if you already have heart disease,
you can halt and even reverse its
progress by following Dr Cutting's simple
steps. Don't be a victim – take action
NOW!

> 'This is an exceptional book.'
> – *Cardiology News*

Stroke – the 'at your fingertips' guide
*Dr Anthony Rudd, Penny Irwin
and Bridget Penhale*   £14.99
This essential guidebook tells you all
about strokes – most importantly how to
recover from them.

As well as providing clear explanations
of the medical processes, tests, and
treatments, the book is full of practical
advice, including recuperation plans; you
will find it inspiring.

> 'An excellent and long overdue
> book.' – *Donal O'Kelly, Director,
> Different Strokes*

Beating Depression – the 'at your fingertips' guide
£14.99
*Dr Stefan Cembrowicz
and Dr Dorcas Kingham*
Depression is one of most common
illnesses in the world – affecting up to one
in four people at some time in their lives.
Beating Depression shows sufferers and
their families that they are not alone, and
offers tried and tested techniques for
overcoming depression.

> 'A sympathetic and understanding
> guide.' – *Marjorie Wallace,
> Chief Executive, SANE*

PRIORITY ORDER FORM

Cut out or photocopy this form and send it (post free in the UK) to:

Class Publishing Priority Service   **Telephone: 01752 202 301**

FREEPOST (PAM 6219)   **Fax: 01752 202 333**

Plymouth PL6 7ZZ

Please send me urgently   *Post included*
(*tick boxes below*)   *price per copy (UK only)*

☐ **High Blood Pressure – the 'at your fingertips' guide**   £17.99
    (ISBN 1 85959 090 X)

☐ **Heart Health – the 'at your fingertips' guide**   £17.99
    (ISBN 1 85959 009 8)

☐ **Stop that heart attack!**   £17.99
    (ISBN 1 85959 096 9)

☐ **Diabetes – the 'at your fingertips' guide**   £17.99
    (ISBN 1 85959 087 X)

☐ **Stroke – the 'at your fingertips' guide**   £17.99
    (ISBN 1 872362 98 2)

☐ **Sexual Health for Men – the 'at your fingertips' guide** £17.99
    (ISBN 1 85959 011 X)

☐ **Beating Depression – the 'at your fingertips' guide**   £17.99
    (ISBN 1 85959 063 2)

                                       TOTAL   _____

Easy ways to pay

Cheque: I enclose a cheque payable to Class Publishing for £ _____

Credit card: Please debit my

        ☐ Mastercard   ☐ Visa   ☐ Amex   ☐ Switch

Number _____ Expiry date _____

Name _____

My address for delivery is _____

_____

Town _____ County _____ Postcode _____

Telephone number (*in case of query*) _____

Credit card billing address if different from above _____

_____

Town _____ County _____ Postcode _____

Class Publishing's guarantee: remember that if, for any reason, you are not satisfied with these books, we will refund all your money, without any questions asked. Prices and VAT rates may be altered for reasons beyond our control.